STUDY GUIDE FOR THE

Core Curriculum for Oncology Nursing

STUDY GUIDE FOR THE
Core Curriculum for Oncology Nursing

THIRD EDITION

Claudette G. Varricchio, RN, DSN, FAAN

Program Director and Nurse Consultant
National Cancer Institute
National Institutes of Health
Bethesda, Maryland

Patricia F. Jassak, RN, MS, AOCN

Administrative Director
Creticos Cancer Center, Illinois Masonic Medical Center
Chicago, Illinois

W.B. SAUNDERS COMPANY
A Division of Harcourt Brace & Company
Philadelphia London Toronto Sydney

W.B. SAUNDERS COMPANY

A Division of Harcourt Brace & Company

The Curtis Center
Independence Square West
Philadelphia, Pennsylvania 19106

NOTICE

Oncology Nursing is an ever-changing field. Standard safety precautions must be followed, but as new research and clinical experience broaden our knowledge, changes in treatment and drug therapy become necessary or appropriate. Readers are advised to check the product information currently provided by the manufacturer of each drug or vaccine to be administered to verify the recommended dose, the method and duration of administration, and contraindications. It is the responsibility of the treating physician relying on experience and knowledge of the patient to determine dosages and the best treatment for the patient. Neither the Publisher nor the author assumes any responsibility for any injury and/or damage to persons or property.

THE PUBLISHER

STUDY GUIDE FOR THE CORE CURRICULUM FOR ONCOLOGY NURSING   ISBN 0-7216-7157-8

Printed in the United States of America

Last digit is the print number: 9   8   7   6   5   4   3   2   1

Contributors

Doris Ahana, RN, MSN, OCN

Oncology Clinical Nurse Specialist, Cancer Rehabilitation Services, and CARES Coordinator, St. Francis Medical Center, Honolulu, Hawaii
Symptom Management and Supportive Care: Rehabilitation and Resources

Joyce Alexander, RN, MSN, AOCN

Clinical Nurse Specialist, Oncology and Bone Marrow Transplant, Halifax Medical Center, Daytona Beach, Florida
Nursing Care of the Client With Lymphoma and Multiple Myeloma

Catherine M. Bender, RN, PhD

Assistant Professor, University of Pittsburgh School of Nursing and University of Pittsburgh Cancer Institute, Pittsburgh, Pennsylvania
Nursing Implications of Antineoplastic Therapy

Marge Bernice, RN-C, MS, OCN

Women's Health Care Nurse Practitioner, The Queen's Medical Center, Honolulu, Hawaii
Nursing Care of the Client With Breast Cancer

Marva Bohen, RN, MS

Manager, Fairview Pain Management Center, Fairview University Medical Center, Riverside Campus, Minneapolis, Minnesota
Nursing Care of the Client With Cancer of the Neurologic System

Jeannine M. Brant, RN, MS, AOCN

Assistant Affiliate Professor, Montana State University, Bozeman; Oncology Clinical Nurse Specialist and Pain Consultant, Saint Vincent Hospital and Health Center, Billings, Montana
Comfort

Lynne Brophy, RN, MSN

Oncology Nurse, Cincinnati Hematology-Oncology, Cincinnati, Ohio
Immunology

Kathleen A. Calzone, RN, MSN

Nursing Coordinator, Cancer Risk Evaluation Program, University of Pennsylvania Cancer Center, Philadelphia, Pennsylvania
Genetics

Dawn Camp-Sorrell, RN, MSN, FNP, AOCN

Oncology Nurse Practitioner, University of Alabama at Birmingham Hospital, Birmingham, Alabama
Myelosuppression

Ellen Carr, RN, MSN, AOCN

Clinical Consultant, San Diego, California
Nursing Care of the Client with Bone and Soft Tissue Cancers; Changes in Oncology Health Care Settings

Mary Ann Crouch, RN, MSN

Clinical Associate, Duke University School of Nursing, Durham; Assistant Chief Operating Officer, Duke University Hospital, Durham, North Carolina
Cancer Economics and Health Care Reform

April J. Dumond, RN, MSN, OCN

Oncology Nursing Educator, Oncology Nursing Associates, Maumelle, Arkansas
Alterations in Nutrition; Alterations in Elimination; Alterations in Ventilation

Coni Ellis, RN-CS, C, MS, CETN, OCN

Adjunct Faculty, School of Nursing, University of Texas Health Science Center, Houston; Nursing Outreach Coordinator and Wound, Ostomy, Continence Program Coordinator, University of Texas M.D. Anderson Cancer Center, Houston, Texas
  Professional Issues in Cancer Care

Jean Ellsworth-Wolk, RN, MS, AOCN

Oncology Nurse Educator/Consultant, Cleveland, Ohio
  Principles of Preparation, Administration, and Disposal of Antineoplastic Agents

Susan A. Ezzone, RN, MS, ANP

Auxiliary Clinical Instructor, The Ohio State University College of Nursing, Columbus; Clinical Nurse Specialist, Arthur G. James Cancer Hospital and Research Institute, The Ohio State University Medical Center, Columbus, Ohio
  Nursing Care of the Client With Leukemia

Joanne Peter Finley, RN, MS

Oncology Nurse Specialist, Potomac, Maryland
  Metabolic Emergencies

Beth A. Freitas, RN, MSN, OCN

Manager, Cancer Institute and Performance Improvement, The Queen's Medical Center, Honolulu, Hawaii
  Coping: Altered Body Image and Alopecia

Patricia M. Grimm, RN, PhD, CS

Associate Professor and American Cancer Society Professor of Oncology Nursing, The Johns Hopkins University School of Nursing; Faculty, Johns Hopkins Oncology Center, Baltimore, Maryland
  Coping: Psychosocial Issues

Mary Magee Gullatte, RN, MN, ANP, AOCN

Nell Hodgson Woodruff School of Nursing, Emory University, Atlanta; Director of Nursing, Oncology and Transplant Nursing, Emory University and Crawford Long Hospitals, Atlanta, Georgia
  Legal Issues Influencing Cancer Care

Jane C. Hunter, RN, MN, ANP

Adult Nurse Practitioner, Community Care Services, Presbyterian Health Care Services, Charlotte, North Carolina
  Structural Emergencies

Joanne K. Itano, RN, PhD, OCN

Associate Professor, University of Hawaii at Manoa School of Nursing, Honolulu, Hawaii
  Cultural Issues

Ryan R. Iwamoto, ARNP, MN, AOCN

Clinical Instructor, School of Nursing, University of Washington, Seattle; Nurse Practitioner/Clinical Nurse Specialist, Department of Radiation Oncology, Virginia Mason Medical Center, Seattle, Washington
  Nursing Care of the Client with Head and Neck Cancer

Patricia F. Jassak, RN, MS, AOCN

Administrative Director, Creticos Cancer Center, Illinois Masonic Medical Center, Chicago, Illinois
  Nursing Care of the Client with HIV-Related Cancer

Mary B. Johnson, RN, PhD, OCN, HNC

Associate Professor, St. Olaf College, Northfield, Minnesota
  The Education Process

Marilyn A. Kline, RN, BSN, OCN

Arizona Urologic Specialists, Tucson, Arizona
  Structural Emergencies

Susan Leigh, RN, BSN

Cancer Survivorship Consultant, Tucson, Arizona
  Coping: Survivorship Issues and Financial Concerns

Julena Lind, RN, PhD

Assistant Professor of Clinical Nursing and Associate Director, Independent Health Professions, University of Southern California, Los Angeles, California
  Nursing Care of the Client with Cancer of the Urinary System; Nursing Care of the Client with Lung Cancer

Alice J. Longman, RN, EdD, FAAN

Professor Emeritus, The University of Arizona College of Nursing, Tucson, Arizona
  Nursing Care of the Client with Skin Cancer

June Lunney, RN, PhD

Program Director, National Institute of Nursing Research, Bethesda, Maryland
  Symptom Management and Supportive Care: Dying and Death

Carolyn S. J. Ma, PharmD

Clinical Pharmacy Specialist in Oncology and Pain Management, The Queen's Medical Center, Honolulu, Hawaii

Symptom Management and Supportive Care: Pharmacologic Interventions

Jan Hawthorne Maxson, RN, MSN, AOCN

Clinical Faculty, Frances Payne Bolton School of Nursing, Case Western Reserve University; Care Manager, Women's Surgical Oncology, University Hospitals of Cleveland, Cleveland, Ohio

Principles of Preparation, Administration, and Disposal of Antineoplastic Agents

Molly J. Moran, RN, MS, CNP

Clinical Nurse Specialist, Arthur G. James Cancer Hospital and Research Institute, The Ohio State University Medical Center, Columbus, Ohio

Nursing Care of the Client with Leukemia

Candis H. Morrison, RN, PhD, ACNP

Associate Professor, The Johns Hopkins University School of Nursing; Nurse Practitioner, The Johns Hopkins Oncology Center, Baltimore, Maryland

Screening and Early Detection of Cancer

Mary Mrozek-Orlowski, ARNP, MSN, AOCN

Adjuvant Faculty, Massachusetts General Hospital Institute of Health, Boston, Massachusetts; Instructor, Dartmouth Medical School, Hanover, New Hampshire; Nurse Practitioner, Comprehensive Breast Care Program, Norris Cotton Cancer Center, Lebanon, New Hampshire

Alterations in Circulation

Patricia W. Nishimoto, RN, MPH, DNS

Associate Professor, University of Hawaii School of Nursing, Honolulu; Adult Oncology Clinical Nurse Specialist, Tripler Army Medical Center, Honolulu, Hawaii

Sexuality

Sharon J. Olsen, RN, MS, AOCN

Assistant Professor, The Johns Hopkins University School of Nursing, Baltimore, Maryland

Prevention of Cancer

Rose Mary Padberg, RN, MA, OCN

Nurse Consultant, Division of Cancer Prevention, National Cancer Institute, Rockville, Maryland

Selected Ethical Issues in Cancer Care

Jennifer Douglas Pearce, RN, MSN, OCN

Associate Professor, Department of Nursing, University of Cincinnati Raymond Walters College, Cincinnati, Ohio

Alterations in Mobility, Skin Integrity, and Neurologic Status

Jan Petree, RN, MS, FNP

Nurse Practitioner, Stanford Health Systems, Stanford, California

Symptom Management and Supportive Care: Therapies and Procedures

Lana Hlava Renaud, RN, MSN, OCN

Research Nurse Coordinator, Illinois Masonic Cancer Center, Chicago, Illinois

Nursing Care of the Client with Genital Cancer

Paula Trahan Rieger, RN, MSN, ANP, CS, OCN, FAAN

Clinical Instructor, The University of Texas Health Science Center School of Nursing; Cancer Detection Specialist, Human Clinical Cancer Genetics Program, The University of Texas M.D. Anderson Cancer Center, Houston, Texas

Nursing Implications of Biotherapy

Paul J. Ross, RN, MA, MSN(c)

Adjunct Instructor, Department of Anthropology, University of Hawaii at Manoa; Oncology RN CNIII, The Queen's Medical Center, Honolulu, Hawaii

Issues and Challenges: Alternative Therapies

Ellen Sitton, RN, MSN, RT(T)

Advanced Practice Nurse, Radiation Oncology and Education, University of Southern California Kenneth Norris Jr. Cancer Hospital, Los Angeles, California

Nursing Implications of Radiation Therapy

Roberta Anne Strohl, RN, MN, AOCN

Clinical Nurse Specialist, Radiation Oncology, University of Maryland, Baltimore, Maryland

Nursing Care of the Client with Cancer of the Gastrointestinal Tract

Thomas J. Szopa, RN, MS, AOCN, CETN

Clinical Nurse Specialist, Oncology and Ostomy/Wound Management, Elliot Hospital, Manchester, New Hampshire

Nursing Implications of Surgical Treatment

Karen N. Taoka, RN, MN, AOCN

Clinical Assistant Professor of Nursing, University of Hawaii at Manoa School of Nursing; Clinical Nurse Specialist, Oncology, The Queen's Medical Center, Honolulu, Hawaii

> *Symptom Management and Supportive Care: Pharmacologic Interventions*

Robi Thomas, RN, MS, AOCN

Oncology Clinical Nurse Specialist, St. Joseph Mercy–Oakland Hospital, Pontiac, Michigan

> *Alterations in Nutrition; Nursing Implications of Bone Marrow and Stem Cell Transplantation*

Deborah Lowe Volker, RN, MA, OCN

Nursing Education Coordinator, The University of Texas M. D. Anderson Cancer Center, Houston, Texas

> *Carcinogenesis; Application of the Standards of Practice and Education*

Reviewers

Mary Ann Anglim, RN, MEd

Assistant Professor, University of Minnesota School of Nursing, Minneapolis, Minnesota

Diane M. Otte, RN, MS, OCN

Alegant Health, Omaha, Nebraska

Margaret Ann Sawin Pierce, RN, MSN, MPH, AOCN

University of Tennessee, Knoxville, Tennessee

Mary Beth Riley, RN, MSN, OCN

Robert Lurie Cancer Center, Northwestern University, Rush Cancer Institute, Chicago, Illinois

Preface

The *Study Guide for the Core Curriculum for Oncology Nursing,* third edition, a companion to the *Core Curriculum for Oncology Nursing,* third edition, is a resource for nurses who want to review a basic level of oncology nursing knowledge. This book may also serve as a reference source of information on oncology nursing topics. Educators may find it useful as a bank of test questions to guide the development of course-related materials.

This book is based on and is intended for use as a companion text to the *Core Curriculum for Oncology Nursing,* third edition. Many of the questions, rationales, and references were written by the authors of the corresponding chapters in the *Core Curriculum* text. The initial and final manuscripts were reviewed by clinical oncology nurses and oncology nurse educators for clinical relevance, accuracy, and clarity. Answers were chosen to reflect national practice trends at the time the text was written and may not reflect some regional clinical practices.

The book is divided into chapters whose content parallels the *Core Curriculum.* Each chapter has multiple choice questions. The correct answer and a rationale for the answer are provided. The *Core Curriculum for Oncology Nursing,* third edition, is the primary source for the text. A list of additional references is provided at the end of each chapter for further study of the content area.

The number of questions on each topic was derived from the percent of questions for that content area established by the Oncology Nursing Certification Corporation in the "Blueprint for the Oncology Nursing Certification Exam" provided to applicants for the certification exam. The subjects covered in both this study guide and in the *Core Curriculum* go beyond those known to be included in the certification exam.

Claudette G. Varricchio
Patricia F. Jassak

Contents

PART **VIII**

Professional Performance, 197

PART I

Quality of Life

Comfort

Jeannine M. Brant

Select the best answer for each of the following questions:

1. Pain is defined as an unpleasant sensory and emotional experience associated with
   A. actual tissue damage.
   B. actual or potential tissue damage.
   C. observable pain behaviors.
   D. physiologic signs and symptoms that the pain exists.

2. Nociceptive pain characteristics include
   A. compression or injury to peripheral, sympathetic, or central nervous system.
   B. radiating and shooting sensations.
   C. activation of nociceptors in deep and cutaneous tissues.
   D. numbness and tingling sensations.

3. A client taking opioids for cancer pain begins to require more medication to provide the same amount of analgesia. This is known as
   A. physical dependence.
   B. drug tolerance.
   C. addiction.
   D. equianalgesia.

4. Physical dependence or drug dependence is which type of phenomenon?
   A. Psychologic.
   B. Physiologic.
   C. Addiction.
   D. Obsessive-compulsive.

5. A client with terminal gastric cancer is admitted in a comatose condition. The spouse states that the client had been taking long-acting morphine 200 mg q8h for the past 6 months. What should the nurse do?
   A. Hold the medication because the client does not appear to be in pain.
   B. Try to give oral morphine tablet hoping it will slip down into the stomach.
   C. Crush the long-acting morphine and give it through a feeding tube.
   D. Notify the physician and ask for an alternative route of administration.

6. The incidence of addiction in clients taking opioid substances is
   A. approximately 10%.
   B. approximately 5%.
   C. approximately 1%.
   D. less than 1%.

7. The most common cause of cancer pain is
   A. spinal cord compression.
   B. peripheral neuropathy.
   C. bone metastases.
   D. abdominal pressure.

8. Which cancer pain syndrome may be an oncologic emergency?
   A. Postmastectomy pain.
   B. Severe back pain.
   C. Peripheral neuropathy.
   D. Mucositis.

3

9. Cancer pain related to plexopathies
   A. often precedes spinal cord compression.
   B. is often followed by extremity weakness and sensory loss.
   C. is a result of immunosuppression related to chemotherapy.
   D. involves interruption of the intercostobrachial nerves.

10. A post-thoracotomy client with complications has been using a meperidine patient-controlled analgesic pump for approximately 2 weeks. What is a possible outcome?
    A. Better pain relief.
    B. Physical withdrawal.
    C. Oversedation.
    D. Seizures and central nervous system toxicity.

11. The classification of adjuvant pain medications recommended for the treatment of metastatic bone pain is
    A. nonsteroidal antiinflammatory agents (NSAIDs).
    B. analeptics.
    C. benzodiazepines.
    D. muscle relaxants.

12. A client with cancer has a pain score of 2 but complains of "always being sleepy." An appropriate intervention would be to recommend to the physician the addition of
    A. amitriptyline.
    B. phenytoin.
    C. methylphenidate (Ritalin).
    D. NSAID.

13. Pediatric pain assessment is performed according to
    A. the chronologic age of the child.
    B. the developmental age of the child.
    C. universal pain faces for all children.
    D. the child's social and psychologic well-being.

14. The temporal assessment of pain includes the
    A. location of the pain.
    B. intensity of the pain.
    C. quality of the pain.
    D. onset and duration of pain.

15. Cancer pain is best managed with the use of
    A. a patient-controlled analgesic pump.
    B. short-acting opioids administered around the clock.
    C. frequent administration of breakthrough medications.
    D. long-acting opioids administered around the clock.

16. Which of the following is the symptom most frequently experienced by the client with cancer?
    A. Fatigue.
    B. Alopecia.
    C. Nausea and vomiting.
    D. Neutropenia.

17. Erythropoietin (rEPO) works by
    A. increasing the oxygen content in the blood, thus increasing hemoglobin.
    B. preventing chemotherapy-induced neutropenia.
    C. stimulating the production of red blood cells.
    D. replacing blood cell components.

18. A client has been unable to bathe independently lately because of being "too tired." Which dimension of the fatigue assessment would reveal this?
    A. Temporal assessment.
    B. Affective assessment.
    C. Cognitive assessment.
    D. Behavioral assessment.

19. To assess the effect of fatigue on a client's cognitive or mental function, ask the client
    A. about sleeping patterns.
    B. to count backwards by 3s beginning at 100.
    C. about the circadian pattern of the fatigue.
    D. about ability to perform ADL.

20. Nursing diagnoses that may be associated with fatigue include all of the following *except*
    A. activity tolerance.
    B. hopelessness.
    C. self-care deficit.
    D. social isolation.

21. A client states fatigue interferes with her ability to keep her house clean, do the laundry, and care for her 2- and 4-year-old girls. These activities are called
    A. emotional aspects of fatigue.
    B. basic activities of daily living.
    C. advanced activities of daily living.
    D. mental wellness activities of daily living.

22. The nurse educates Mrs. Smith about interventions that conserve energy. They include all of the following *except*
    A. prioritizing needs.
    B. modifying plans if needed.
    C. attending an aerobic class to promote the body's energy regulatory system.
    D. pacing her schedule.

23. Which of the following actions have clients found to be helpful in combating fatigue?
    A. Reduction of usual lifestyle activities.
    B. Increased fat in the diet.
    C. Participation in mild exercise such as walking, golf, or swimming.
    D. Performance of daily chores, cooking, and cleaning before other activities.

24. Cancer-related conditions that typically cause pruritus include all of the following *except*
    A. leukemia and Hodgkin's disease.
    B. dehydration.
    C. infection.
    D. alopecia.

25. Potential laboratory findings associated with pruritus include
    A. elevated white blood cell count.
    B. hypouricemia.
    C. anemia.
    D. decreased creatinine.

26. A client received adjuvant chemotherapy for breast cancer last week. She now presents in the office with a complaint of pruritus. The assessment for pruritus would include all of the following *except* the presence of
    A. scratch marks, erythema, and skin dryness.
    B. urea on the skin.
    C. nausea, vomiting, and constipation.
    D. stress and anxiety.

27. The nurse instructs the client to modify the environment to minimize pruritus by
    A. keeping room humidity high.
    B. keeping the room temperature warm.
    C. using silk sheets.
    D. staying outdoors as much as possible.

28. The nurse recommends that the client maximize comfort while experiencing pruritus by all of the following *except*
    A. cutting nails short and clean to scratch the pruritic areas.
    B. medicated baths with antipruritics.
    C. local anesthetic creams.
    D. massaging the pruritic areas.

29. An inflammatory reaction occurring in previously irradiated tissue often associated with dry desquamation and pruritus is also known as
    A. radiation enhancement.
    B. radiation recall.
    C. inflammation of keratoses.
    D. acral erythema.

30. The client is hospitalized with acute myelogenous leukemia. Septicemia develops and an antibiotic regimen is started. Immediately a trunk rash with pruritus develops. Interventions may include all of the following *except*
    A. administering antihistamines.
    B. notifying the physician and obtaining an order for an alternative antibiotic.
    C. administering corticosteroids.
    D. increasing antihistamines in the morning as pruritus frequently increases during the daytime.

31. Risk factors for sleep disorder include all of the following *except*
    A. presence of pain, pruritus, and other concurrent symptoms.
    B. delirium, confusion, and altered mental status.
    C. increased estrogen levels from chemotherapy.
    D. paraneoplastic syndromes with associated increase in corticosteroid levels.

32. A client with recently diagnosed myeloma complains of being unable to go to sleep. What

bedtime routine advice should the nurse provide?

A. Promote relaxation 2 hours before bedtime.
B. Drink a glass of wine or alcohol at bedtime.
C. Participate in an exercise activity before bedtime to promote exhaustion.
D. Begin taking a sleeping aid.

33. A sleep assessment normally includes all *except*
A. usual pattern of sleep.
B. client's sleeping environment including noise and light factors.
C. the impact of insomnia on daily living.
D. an exercise tolerance test.

34. Physical signs of sleep deprivation include
A. dark circles under the eyes, nystagmus, incorrect word usage.
B. dark circles under the eyes, overpronunciation of words, and a loud voice.
C. stuttering, nystagmus, and loss of balance.
D. slurred speech, a loud voice, and an impaired gait.

NOTES

ANSWERS

1. *Answer:* B
Rationale: Pain is a warning of actual or potential tissue damage.

2. *Answer:* C
Rationale: Nociceptive pain refers to the stimulation or activation of nociceptors (pain fibers) in deep and cutaneous tissues such as the skin, bone, and thoracic and abdominal organs.

3. *Answer:* B
Rationale: Tolerance means that after repeated administration of a narcotic, a given dosage begins to lose its effectiveness; it begins to have a shorter duration of action and then less analgesic action. This is a physiologic phenomenon that clients cannot control.

4. *Answer:* B
Rationale: Physical dependence is a physiologic phenomenon that occurs after repeated administration of an opioid. Withdrawal symptoms occur when the narcotic is not taken. This will occur if the client has been taking opioids for an extended time.

5. *Answer:* D
Rationale: The client will likely experience withdrawal if the morphine is withheld. Crushing the tablet will interfere with the sustained-release action of the drug. The best solution is to notify the physician and give the drug by an alternate route.

6. *Answer:* D
Rationale: Studies show that fewer than 1% of clients experience the psychologic phenomenon of addiction while taking opioids for pain relief. Addiction is an overwhelming involvement with obtaining and using a drug for psychologic reasons.

7. *Answer:* C
Rationale: Bone metastases occur in the most common neoplasms such as cancer of the breast, prostate, and lung. Pain is almost always associated with bone destruction or compression of the nerves and soft tissue by the bone.

8. *Answer:* B
Rationale: One of the earliest signs of spinal cord compression is severe back pain. Cord compression may result in permanent paralysis and neurologic deficits and is therefore an oncologic emergency.

9. *Answer:* B
Rationale: Plexopathies occur when cervical, brachial, and lumbosacral nerves are infiltrated or compressed. The nerve compression causes pain followed by extremity weakness and sensory loss.

10. *Answer:* D
Rationale: Meperidine contains a metabolite called "normeperidine," which accumulates in the body and lowers the seizure and central nervous system toxicity symptoms such as twitching.

11. *Answer:* A
Rationale: NSAIDs block prostaglandins, pain-producing neurotransmitters that occur with bone metastasis.

12. *Answer:* C
Rationale: Analeptics such as ritalin may counteract sedation and may improve quality of life.

13. *Answer:* B
Rationale: Children are highly variable by age and social condition. The only way to accurately assess a child is by his or her developmental age.

14. *Answer:* D
Rationale: Temporality refers to how the pain changes over time and includes the onset, duration, exacerbating, and relieving factors of pain.

15. *Answer:* D
Rationale: Scheduled long-acting opioids provide a therapeutic blood level of analgesia and prevent "peaks and troughs" during the pain experience.

16. *Answer:* A
Rationale: Fatigue occurs in almost 100% of clients with cancer. It is a common symptom of cancer and all cancer therapies.

17. *Answer:* C
Rationale: The use of rEPO stimulates the production of red blood cells.

18. *Answer:* D
Rationale: The behavioral assessment reveals how the fatigue affects the client's ability to perform activities of daily living.

19. *Answer:* B
Rationale: The cognitive or mental dimension of fatigue involves the assessment of concentration, memory, and alertness; counting backward by 3s is an example.

20. *Answer:* A
Rationale: The client would experience activity intolerance with fatigue.

21. *Answer:* C
Rationale: Bathing, grooming, dressing, and mobility are considered basic activities of daily living, whereas housekeeping, shopping, laundry, child care, and work are more advanced activities of daily living.

22. *Answer:* C
Rationale: Although exercise may promote the body's energy, this is not an intervention that conserves energy.

23. *Answer:* C
Rationale: Trying to maintain a normal lifestyle is important, and participation in mild exercise may promote energy. Protein and carbohydrate intake should be increased, and daily activities should be prioritized for each individual.

24. *Answer:* D
Rationale: Alopecia typically begins with a tender head followed by hair loss but is not associated with pruritus.

25. *Answer:* A
Rationale: An elevated white blood cell count may signify infection that may cause pruritus. The patient with pruritus may experience hyperuricemia and an increased creatinine level.

26. *Answer:* C
Rationale: The presence of nausea, vomiting, and constipation would not likely lead to pruritus. The skin assessment reveals how the client is coping with the pruritus. Hyperuricemia can stimulate pruritus; stress and anxiety may also precipitate pruritus.

27. *Answer:* A
Rationale: Pruritus is minimized by increasing room humidity, preventing vasodilation by keeping the room temperature cool, and using cotton sheets and clothing and hypoallergenic soaps.

28. *Answer:* A
Rationale: Scratching pruritic areas with the fingernails may cause the skin to break down and become infected. Massaging or rubbing the area is a safer alternative.

29. *Answer:* B
Rationale: Radiation recall with associated pruritus often occurs if chemotherapy, especially doxorubicin and dactinomycin, is administered simultaneously or close to radiation therapy.

30. *Answer:* D
Rationale: All interventions are appropriate except that pruritus frequently increases at night.

31. *Answer:* C
Rationale: Interrupted sleep patterns may be caused by low estrogen levels triggered by menopause, which may or may not be related to cancer therapies.

32. *Answer:* A
Rationale: Relaxation before bedtime is important both physically and mentally. Alcohol may be a stimulant and interfere with sleep, whereas exercise should be performed earlier. Bedtime routine adjustment should be tried before a sleeping aid.

33. *Answer:* D
Rationale: Exercise is often not a factor in sleep disorders. Other parameters including a psychosocial assessment are encouraged.

34. *Answer:* A

Rationale: Dark circles under the eyes, nystagmus, incorrect word usage, slurred speech, frequent yawning, and ptosis of the eyelids are all physical signs of sleep deprivation. Stuttering and a loud voice are not usually associated with sleep disorders.

BIBLIOGRAPHY

American Pain Society. (1992). *Principles of Analgesic Use in the Treatment of Acute Pain and Chronic Cancer Pain* (3rd ed.). Skokie, IL: Author.

Brant, J., Brumit, J., Forseth, J., et al. (1996). *Pain and Symptom Management in the Terminally Ill.* Billings, MT: Big Sky Hospice.

Brant, J.M. (1998). Comfort. In J.K. Itano, K. N. Taoka (eds.). *Core Curriculum for Oncology Nursing* (3rd ed.). Philadelphia: WB Saunders, pp. 3–29.

Breitbart, W., Bruera, E., Chochivov, H., et al. (1995). Neuropsychiatric syndromes and psychological symptoms in patients with advanced cancer. *J Pain Symptom Manage 10*(2), 131–141.

Collins, J.J., Grier, H.E., Kinney, H.C., et al. (1995). Control of severe pain in children with terminal malignancy. *J Pediatr 126,* 653–657.

DeSpain, J.D. (1992). Dermatologic toxicity. In M.C. Perry (ed.). *The Chemotherapy Source Book.* Baltimore: Williams & Wilkins, pp. 531–547.

Glaus, A. (1993). Assessment of fatigue in cancer and non-cancer patients and in healthy individuals. *Supportive Care in Cancer 1*(6), 305–315.

Graydon, J.E., Bubela, N., Irvine, D., et al. (1995). Fatigue-reducing strategies used by patients receiving treatment for cancer. *Cancer Nurs 18*(1), 23–28.

Irvine, D.M., Vincent, L., Graydon, J.E., et al. (1994). The prevalence and correlates of fatigue in patients receiving treatment with chemotherapy and radiotherapy. *Cancer Nurs 17*(5), 367–378.

Jacox, A., Carr, D.B., Payne, R., et al. (1994). *Management of Cancer Pain, Clinical Practice Guideline No. 9.* Rockville, MD: AHCPR.

Richardson, A. (1995). Fatigue in cancer patients: A review of the literature. *Eur J Cancer Care 4*(1), 20–32.

Watson, C.P.N. (1994). Antidepressant drugs as adjuvant analgesics. *J Pain Symptom Manage 9*(6), 392–405.

NOTES

2

Coping: Psychosocial Issues

Patricia M. Grimm

Select the best answer for each of the following questions:

1. In considering what places a client with cancer at risk for emotional distress, which one of the following factors can be influenced by nursing interventions?
   A. Disruption of age-specific developmental life tasks.
   B. Lack of prognostic certainty.
   C. Knowledge of cancer diagnosis, treatment, and expected outcomes.
   D. Prior life experiences and coping ability.

2. In response to a diagnosis of ineffective individual coping, the nurse might choose all of the following interventions *except*
   A. evaluation, with the client, of the effectiveness of current coping strategies.
   B. instruction in relaxation, imagery, and other holistic stress reduction techniques.
   C. providing referrals as needed to the psychiatric liaison nurse, psychologist, social worker.
   D. strengthening the client's social support system.

3. While administering chemotherapy to a young woman, you observe that both she and her husband appear quite anxious. Which of the following responses would be considered an *inappropriate* response in dealing with their anxiety?
   A. I realize that this experience can be very upsetting. I will tell you about each step of the procedure, and you can keep me informed about your concerns.
   B. I will teach you more about this procedure later, but for now you can observe what I am doing and ask questions as you like.
   C. You both appear to be quite anxious. Do you have questions or concerns that you want to discuss before we start?
   D. You seem concerned. Trust me, I have done this hundreds of times. You can both relax, and I will be done in a minute.

4. Mrs. R. is a 76-year-old retired banker who has done well for 2 years after pelvic exenteration. Recently she experienced a recurrence. She now has multiple draining fistulae and has been told that she is not a candidate for further treatment. Her son said that her response has been complete withdrawal. She has changed from a meticulous dresser and housekeeper to neglecting both. She refuses to eat and blames herself for not going for regular Pap smears. She refuses help from her son, saying he is "wasting his time, I deserve to die." Her responses reflect developmental, situational, and disease-related characteristics *most* suggestive of
   A. fear of death.
   B. low self-esteem.
   C. neurotic anxiety.
   D. role abandonment.

5. Mrs. R. was hospitalized for management of the fistulae. Once the drainage was managed ef-

fectively, Mrs. R. seemed to show more interest in her care. During this phase, the most therapeutic nursing approach to facilitate adaptive behavior would be to

    A. initiate a referral for rehabilitative counseling.

    B. make no demands on Mrs. R. for her own care.

    C. positively reinforce Mrs. R.'s approaches to self-care.

    D. transfer responsibility for Mrs. R.'s care to her family.

6. The nursing plan included a referral to a client-to-client visitation program to assist Mrs. R. in adapting to the life changes imposed by the progression of her cancer. Which of the following would provide this service?

    A. CanSurMount.

    B. I Can Cope.

    C. National Cancer Institute.

    D. Reach to Recovery.

7. All of the following factors may place a cancer client at risk for symptoms of anxiety *except*

    A. excessive intake of caffeine or nicotine.

    B. experiencing intensive therapies, such as mutilating surgery or bone marrow transplantation (BMT).

    C. increasing activity and exercise.

    D. treatment with corticosteriods, neuroleptic antiemetics.

8. Mr. L. is admitted to an oncology unit and assessment reveals flushed skin, sweating, jerky hand movements, and asking questions repeatedly. The most probable nursing diagnosis would be which of the following?

    A. Anxiety.

    B. Fear.

    C. Low self-esteem.

    D. Phobias.

9. Mr. L. has started taking an antianxiety drug. He tells you that he feels much calmer but that his mouth is so uncomfortably dry that he is thinking about discontinuing the drug. The most therapeutic response would be to

    A. assure him that the dry mouth is not as bad as the anxiety.

    B. call the physician and request an order for another antianxiety drug.

    C. explain that the dryness generally diminishes; increase fluid intake.

    D. support him in his decision and hold the daily dose.

10. Mr. L. also expresses interest in nonpharmacologic approaches to managing his anxiety. In discussing relaxation and guided imagery with him, all of the following are true *except*

    A. guided imagery can give you a sense of control over your present situation.

    B. guided imagery is a form of hypnosis and you will lose consciousness.

    C. muscle tension is part of anxiety; in relaxing your muscles, anxiety is reduced.

    D. practicing these techniques is important to their success.

11. Antianxiety drugs are not discontinued abruptly because a possible withdrawal effect is

    A. hypertensive episodes.

    B. narcolepsy.

    C. seizures.

    D. severe depression.

12. In admitting a person with cancer whose physical and psychosocial evaluation reflects an anxious state bordering panic, the most therapeutic approach is to be

    A. authoritative and decisive, enunciating clearly.

    B. detached and objective, minimizing patient fears.

    C. thorough and informative, validating knowledge.

    D. supportive and direct, using soothing voice tones.

13. Mrs. S. is admitted to the hospital for the evaluation of metastatic disease related to her diagnosis of breast cancer. Her family is concerned about recent changes in her behavior, i.e., crying, lack of interest in her appearance, changes in sleeping and eating. In considering a referral for evaluation of depression in this patient, it is most important to assess

    A. effect of behavior on family members.

    B. meaning of the illness to the client.

    C. presence of suicidal thoughts.

    D. mental status as an indicator of delirium.

14. Which of the following risk factors for development of depressive symptoms is most amenable to direct nursing interventions?
   A. Family developmental and situational crises.
   B. Inadequate social support.
   C. Inadequate symptom control.
   D. Client history of suicidal thoughts.

15. Physical findings most descriptive of a depressed state include
   A. facial pallor, tense posturing, vocal tremors, and diaphoresis.
   B. flat affect, lack of spontaneity, minimal eye contact, and slumped posture.
   C. inappropriate affect, disheveled dress, sweaty hands, and tremors.
   D. labile emotions, hyperactivity, sighing respirations, and overtalkativeness.

16. Which of the following responses by the nurse would be *most* therapeutic in helping the client deal with the somatic complaints often associated with depression?
   A. Advising the client to minimize these symptoms, thus conserving energy to fight the disease.
   B. Explaining that the symptoms are not "real" and, therefore, need no treatment.
   C. Listening nonjudgmentally and trying diversional techniques as a possible method of alleviation.
   D. Validating that symptoms do or do not have a physiologic basis and providing prompt treatment or placebos for relief.

17. In teaching management of the side effects of antidepressant medication, which of the following would be *most* important for an elderly client?
   A. Change from a lying to a standing position slowly.
   B. Monitor changes in visual acuity.
   C. Increase fluid intake.
   D. Take medication at bedtime.

18. Mr. G. returns to the oncology clinic for treatment of recurrent lymphoma after BMT. He tells you that it is hard to believe that there is a purpose to his experiences, tearfully stating, "I'm really angry and I don't trust anything anymore." The most probable nursing diagnosis would be
   A. anxiety.
   B. ineffective individual coping.

   C. self-esteem disturbance.
   D. spiritual distress.

19. From your past contact with Mr. G., you know him to be a deeply spiritual person, attending church and using prayer to manage the demands of his illness and treatment. Today he angrily refuses when you volunteer to call his pastor for him. Your *best* response to this would be
   A. Getting angry with God isn't going to help.
   B. Perhaps you'd like to tell me more about what you're feeling right now.
   C. Sounds like you'd like some privacy, I'll be back soon.
   D. Would you like me to pray with you?

20. In considering barriers that influence a client's ability to continue his or her spiritual beliefs and practices, the most significant one is
   A. activity and dietary restrictions.
   B. ignorance of health care providers.
   C. lack of privacy.
   D. treatment regimen requirements.

21. An individual's response to the loss of personal control depends on all of the following *except*
   A. duration of time since diagnosis.
   B. individual patterns of coping.
   C. meaning of the loss.
   D. response of family and friends.

22. Mr. J., a 48-year-old businessman, has recently had a diagnosis of lung cancer. He stated, "I don't feel like I have any control over what is happening to me." Which of the following is an appropriate statement for the nurse to make?
   A. Ask your doctor about your care and he will answer your questions.
   B. Ask your wife to let you do more things for yourself.
   C. Let's spend some time talking about your feelings.
   D. We will develop a routine schedule for your care so you will know what to expect.

23. Nursing interventions designed to facilitate Mr. J.'s sense of personal control would include all of the following *except*
   A. asking family to make decisions regarding burdensome areas of treatment and care.

B. discussing with him his feelings regarding personal control.

C. encourage identification of areas over which control can be maintained.

D. provide successful management of symptoms.

24. A behavior that would indicate a need for immediate professional assistance (mental health professional) with Mr. J. is

A. inability to perform activities of daily living.

B. noncompliance with treatment regimen.

C. refusal to discuss personal feelings.

D. verbalization of self-harm intentions.

25. Grief is defined as changes in thinking, feeling, and behaving that occur in response to

A. death of a significant other.

B. disease with an uncertain prognosis.

C. losses related to the aging process.

D. loss of a valued object or person.

26. In discussing the process of grief with clients or family members, all of the following points are correct *except*

A. one's grief response will be influenced by past experiences with loss and grief.

B. reactions that occur more than 1 year after the loss are considered dysfunctional grief.

C. somatic symptoms of grief often occur.

D. specific stages of grief exist.

27. Resolution of the grief process may be facilitated by which of the following interventions?

A. Encouraging discussion of the feelings related to the loss.

B. Discouraging expression of negative feelings, such as anger.

C. Providing sedation as suggested by others.

D. Restricting visitors to family members only.

28. All of the following are grief responses indicative of the need for mental health intervention *except*

A. oversedation.

B. preoccupation with lost object/person.

C. substance abuse.

D. withdrawal or social isolation.

29. Which of the following client responses is *most* representative of a dysfunctional grief response?

A. A 76-year-old man who cared for his wife during the terminal phases of colon cancer reports frequent vivid dreams about his wife and himself.

B. A mother who cries continuously and keeps saying, "No, he can't die," as she attends her 21-year-old son who is dying of leukemia.

C. A 35-year-old woman who, at 6 weeks after a mastectomy, avoids hugs and physical contact with family and friends and has not allowed her husband to look at the surgical site.

D. A 35-year-old widower who prides himself on keeping all of his wife's possessions and visiting her grave daily for the 5 years since her death while neglecting his other responsibilities.

30. Social functioning requires an individual or family to have all of the following *except*

A. ability to problem solve.

B. effective interaction with one's environment.

C. effective reality testing.

D. intact family structure.

31. Ms P., an 18-year-old with a recent diagnosis of leukemia, comes to the clinic for evaluation and determination of treatment. In your assessment of Ms P., you determine that she has lived on her own this past year and has a conflictual relationship with her parents. As you continue your assessment, which additional finding might be indicative of a potential for social dysfunction?

A. Admits she has a temper and has "gotten in trouble before."

B. Has two roommates who accompany her to the clinic.

C. Lives in a community with ethnic and cultural characteristics similar to her own.

D. Seems knowledgeable about her illness and its treatment.

32. Ms P. is admitted to the hospital for induction chemotherapy. Her parents come to visit regularly and often their visits end with angry

shouting matches. As Ms P.'s nurse, you schedule a meeting with the family. Given the above, your initial interventions are directed at

A. assisting family members to discuss their thoughts and feeling about Ms P.'s illness.
B. establishing limits on problematic behavior.
C. instruction regarding the disease and treatment regimen.
D. referral of family to appropriate resources.

33. Ms P. will be discharged soon and will need to move home with her parents for a period of time. In preparing Ms P. for discharge, the following interventions are important *except*

A. encourage Ms P. to participate in self-care.
B. encourage family to limit social contacts and activities.
C. plan for ongoing evaluation of effects of caring on caregiver.
D. provide client and family with skills required for day-to-day care.

NOTES

ANSWERS

1. *Answer:* C
Rationale: Client teaching will help with anxiety and fears. Interventions are not likely to affect other choices.

2. *Answer:* D.
Rationale: Although the nurse may help the client to identify the current social support system, only the client can determine the need to, or ways in which to, strengthen it.

3. *Answer:* D
Rationale: Response A represents a therapeutic response that acknowledges and reassures. B is also therapeutic in that it is nondemanding. C acknowledges anxiety. Response D negates the feelings of the client and spouse, which is a nontherapeutic approach.

4. *Answer:* B
Rationale: Self-negation and self-blame are the defining characteristics that differentiate between low self-esteem and the other mood states.

5. *Answer:* C
Rationale: A is premature, based on the information given. B does not facilitate adaptive behavior. D fosters dependency. C is a behavioral approach that reinforces the desired behavior and is therefore the best response.

6. *Answer:* A
Rationale: I Can Cope is educational; NCI is for research, and Reach to Recovery is for mastectomy clients. CanSurMount is a client visitation program for all types of cancer.

7. *Answer:* C
Rationale: Exercise can actually aid in the management of anxiety symptoms. Other choices place the individual at increased risk.

8. *Answer:* A
Rationale: The stimulus is diffuse, thereby ruling out fear and phobias. Self-negation is not included, thus ruling out response C (low self-esteem).

9. *Answer:* C
Rationale: C represents knowledge of the reactions to the drug and a definitive strategy to al-

leviate. A negates the feelings of the client. B is premature or not indicated. D may lead to symptoms of withdrawal.

10. *Answer:* B
Rationale: A, C, and D are accurate statements. Although sometimes described as self-hypnosis, use of imagery does not result in a loss of consciousness.

11. *Answer:* C
Rationale: Withdrawal symptoms similar in character to those noted with barbiturates and alcohol have been reported after abrupt discontinuation of antianxiety drugs.

12. *Answer:* D
Rationale: During times of intense anxiety, clients benefit most from a supportive environment in which stimuli are limited (e.g., soothing voice, limited information).

13. *Answer:* D
Rationale: It is important to assess for delirium with this client who may be experiencing behavior changes related to metastatic disease. A, B, and C, are valid considerations, but organic causes of behavior must be ruled out first.

14. *Answer:* C
Rationale: Crises and social support can be affected by interventions, but the nurse has limited control of these. Although a history of suicidal thoughts is important to consider, direct interventions to enhance symptom control, particularly pain, may have a more direct effect on depressive symptoms.

15. *Answer:* B
Rationale: Question requires differentiation between depression (B), anxiety (A), psychosis (C), and panic (D).

16. *Answer:* C
Rationale: When there is no physiologic basis for the symptoms, "treatment" of somatic aspects of depression is contraindicated because such actions reinforce these maladaptive behaviors and symptoms. To ask the client to "buck

up" is asking the impossible and instilling guilt. The symptoms are "real" to the client, and diversion may help.

17. *Answer:* A
   Rationale: Risk for falls is a primary concern with an older client. B may or may not be necessary. C is recommended. D depends on the specific drug being taken.

18. *Answer:* D
   Rationale: Loss of purpose, beliefs, and trust is indicative of spiritual distress. Anxiety symptoms are not present, ineffective individual coping is not specific enough, and the client is not exhibiting any self-negating behavior indicative of self-esteem problems.

19. *Answer:* B
   Rationale: B is a therapeutic response and acknowledges the client's discomfort. A denies his feelings. C indicates nurse's discomfort. D is imposing nurse's beliefs.

20. *Answer:* B
   Rationale: The nurse's lack of knowledge can be the most significant barrier. Once we understand beliefs and practices, we can then, it is hoped, consider and explain A, C, and D.

21. *Answer:* A
   Rationale: Loss of personal control can occur at any point in the cancer trajectory.

22. *Answer:* C
   Rationale: Use an open-ended statement to elicit individual perceptions of the response without jumping to conclusions of a diagnosis of loss of personal control.

23. *Answer:* A
   Rationale: To facilitate personal control, the client needs to be included in all decisions regarding treatment and care.

24. *Answer:* D
   Rationale: Statements of suicidal intentions require immediate response for further assessment by a mental health professional. A or B requires problem solving by care providers, and C may be the client's choice.

25. *Answer:* D
   Rationale: All of the situations given may precipitate the grief process, but the best definition of grief is response D.

26. *Answer:* B
   Rationale: A commonly held assumption, but each individual grieves on his or her own timetable. Grief responses are not uncommon more than a year after the loss. The nature of the response, not time, can be the issue.

27. *Answer:* A
   Rationale: Responses other than A represent strategies that block grief work and resolution of the loss.

28. *Answer:* B
   Rationale: Considered a normal aspect of grief response.

29. *Answer:* D
   Rationale: Responses A, B, and C represent normal grief responses. Response D is the best answer because of the evidence of a prolonged and unresolved grief process.

30. *Answer:* D
   Rationale: Although important, individuals without an intact family structure are able to function socially.

31. *Answer:* A
   Rationale: A history of violence and possible legal difficulties may place her at risk. Other data indicate social functioning.

32. *Answer:* A
   Rationale: Although limit setting (B) is appropriate, the first goal would be to better understand this family's emotional issues. Other interventions, while appropriate, do not address the identified problem.

33. *Answer:* B
   Rationale: It is important for client and family to maintain social contacts and activities; therefore do not advise otherwise.

BIBLIOGRAPHY

Belcher, A.E. (1987). Communication with patient and family/significant others. In C. Ziegfeld (ed.). *Core*

Curriculum for Oncology Nursing. Philadelphia: WB Saunders, pp. 347–351.

Carpenito, L.J. (1993). *Nursing Diagnosis: Application to Clinical Practice* (5th ed.). Philadelphia: JB Lippincott.

Carson, V. (1989). *Spiritual Dimensions of Nursing Practice.* Philadelphia: WB Saunders.

Chochinov, H. (1993). Management of grief in the cancer setting. In W. Breitbart & J. Holland (eds.). *Psychiatric Aspects of Symptom Management in Cancer Patients.* Washington, DC: American Psychiatric Press, pp. 231–241.

Fincannon, J. (1995). Analysis of psychiatric referrals and interventions in an oncology population. *Oncol Nurs Forum 22*(1), 87–92.

Germino, B., & O'Rourke, M. (1996). Cancer and the family. In R. McCorkle, M. Grant, M. Frank-Stromborg, & S. Baird (eds). *Cancer Nursing: A Comprehensive Textbook* (2nd ed.). Philadelphia: WB Saunders, pp. 81–92.

Given, B., & Given, C.W. (1996). Family caregiver burden from cancer care. In R. McCorkle, M. Grant, M. Frank-Stromborg, & S. Baird (eds.). *Cancer Nursing: A Comprehensive Textbook* (2nd ed.). Philadelphia: WB Saunders, pp. 93–109.

Grimm, P. (1998). Coping: Psychological issues. In J. Itano & K. Taoka (eds.). *Core Curriculum for Oncology Nursing* (3rd ed.). Philadelphia: WB Saunders, pp. 30–53.

Holland, J. (1990). Clinical course of cancer. In J. Holland & J. Rowland (eds.). *Handbook of Psychooncology: Psychological Care of the Patient with Cancer.* New York: Oxford University Press, pp. 75–100.

Lev, E., Robinson, L., & McCorkle, R. (1996). Loss and bereavement. In R. McCorkle, M. Grant, M. Frank-Stromborg, & S. Baird (eds.). *Cancer Nursing: A Comprehensive Textbook* (2nd ed.). Philadelphia: WB Saunders, pp. 110–118.

McCloskey, J., & Bulechek, G. (1996). *Nursing Interventions Classification (NIC)* (2nd ed.). Baltimore: Mosby.

Townsend, M. (1996). *Psychiatric Mental Health Nursing: Concepts of Care* (2nd ed.). Philadelphia: FA Davis Company.

Valente, S., Saunders, J., & Cohen, M. (1994). Evaluating depression among patients with cancer. *Cancer Prac 2*(1), 65.

NOTES

3

Coping: Altered Body Image and Alopecia

Beth A. Freitas

Select the best answer for each of the following questions:

1. Persons with body image disturbances are frequently found to exhibit self-destructive behavior. In dealing with such behavior the primary goal of the nurse is to assist the client to identify
   A. moral implications of the behavior.
   B. psychologic basis for behavior.
   C. logical basis for behavior.
   D. adverse effects of the behavior.

2. Which of the following client outcome behaviors represents the highest level of adaptation to body image changes?
   A. Discusses changes in body structure and function.
   B. Lists emergency resources to deal with self-destructive behavior.
   C. Serves as a volunteer in a client-to-client visitation program.
   D. Discusses plans to return to previous work role.

3. The predominant fear for an adolescent female with a diagnosis of sarcoma of the tibia to be treated with amputation is
   A. hospitalization.
   B. disfigurement.
   C. desertion.
   D. loss of status.

4. A primary objective of a client visit by a trained volunteer who has adjusted successfully to a similar experience, e.g., Reach to Recovery program for mastectomy clients, is to promote adaptation to changes in
   A. prognosis and life expectancy by discussing the similarity of the visitor's and client's disease.
   B. body structure and functioning by discussing prostheses, clothing, and appearance.
   C. role functioning and lifestyle by discussing vocational rehabilitation and other services available.
   D. sexual and social functioning by discussing personal changes in sexual or social functioning.

5. A client had a colostomy 48 hours ago. Which of the following is *not* an immediate concern regarding his body-image changes?
   A. Refusal to look at surgical area.
   B. Neglect of bathing self.
   C. Not responding to calls from family.
   D. Refusing to get out of bed.

6. Nurses can assist clients in the acceptance of a changed body image. Which of the following nursing interventions is the most supportive?
   A. Stressing a time frame to grieve and then quickly move on.
   B. Facilitating conversations between client and long-lost family.
   C. Educating family immediately regarding body image changes.
   D. Allowing ventilation of negative emotions, especially anger and guilt.

7. Although the body image impact of a treatment differs with each individual, the most significant impact can be seen in which client?
    A. Female mandibulectomy.
    B. Male colostomy.
    C. Female mastectomy.
    D. Male lobectomy.

8. Which of the following strategies is helpful to a daughter's adjustment when her mother has breast cancer?
    A. Inform children about the specifics of the illness.
    B. Have other family members inform the children.
    C. Inform children when the disease outcome is known, about a year after diagnosis.
    D. Keep a structured communication style in place.

9. Which of the following interventions is *not* appropriate to reduce the rate of hair loss?
    A. Sleep on satin pillow.
    B. Use of heated rollers.
    C. Use of cream rinse.
    D. Use of soft-bristle hair brush.

10. The most accurate estimate of the usual hair regrowth is
    A. 1 to 2 weeks after completion of chemotherapy.
    B. 4 to 6 weeks after completion of chemotherapy.
    C. 2 to 4 months after completion of chemotherapy.
    D. 6 to 7 months after completion of chemotherapy.

11. Which of the following statements is correct in regard to chemotherapy-induced alopecia?
    A. Eyelashes and nasal hair are spared.
    B. Type of drug administered affects severity of hair loss.
    C. Administration of multiple drugs decreases severity of alopecia.
    D. Hair loss is usually permanent.

12. Which of the following is considered a common side effect of paclitaxel (Taxol)?
    A. Constipation.
    B. Nausea.
    C. Hair loss.
    D. Fatigue.

13. Which of the following treatments is most likely to cause permanent hair loss?
    A. MOPP therapy for Hodgkin's disease.
    B. 6000 cGy radiation for brain tumor.
    C. CMF for breast cancer.
    D. High-dose ARA-C for leukemia.

14. Client teaching for individuals receiving high doses of chemotherapy drugs should include which of the following suggestions?
    A. Hair loss occurs slowly; therefore adequate time will be available to make plans once the loss begins to occur.
    B. Hair texture and color will be the same as before any loss occurs; therefore wigs should closely resemble original hair.
    C. Hair loss is likely; therefore the best match and the best time psychologically for a wig purchase may be before therapy.
    D. Hair appears thicker with a permanent or with a color application; therefore hair should be permed or colored to lessen evidence of possible hair loss.

ANSWERS

1. *Answer:* D
   Rationale: The adverse effects of body-image disturbances have implications for client safety and should be given priority. Attention to adverse effects is a response that can be an independent nursing role. Other responses refer to interventions that are not necessarily appropriate or are representative of the role of other health professionals.

2. *Answer:* C
   Rationale: C represents actual, rather than planned, reintegration with constructive channeling of energies. Therefore C represents a higher level of adaptation than attention to safety (B), knowledge (A), or planned activity (D).

3. *Answer:* B
   Rationale: Body image is crucial in adolescents.

4. *Answer:* B
   Rationale: Response B delineates the limits of the volunteer's role. Prognosis, personal diseases, or sexual counseling are beyond the scope of responsibility for volunteers.

5. *Answer:* D
   Rationale: Responses A, B, and C are more related to the client's perception of self. Response D is more likely related to the fear of pain with movement versus body image.

6. *Answer:* D
   Rationale: Nurses often find it more difficult to allow clients to express their anger or guilt, but at this point in a client's recovery it may be the most supportive role. Response A is not accurate because grief has no time frame. Response B is not accurate because body image is not affected by this role. Response C is not accurate because this is a preoperative role, and knowledge is not congruent with acceptance.

7. *Answer:* A.
   Rationale: Women have a more negative body image than men in regard to surgical mutilation. Because of the cultural impact of looking perfect, a facial malformation is more difficult to "hide" from society.

8. *Answer:* A
   Rationale: Response B is inappropriate because the client should communicate with the children. Likewise, answers C and D are not correct because communication about the effects of disease should be done within 1 year and the communication style should be open.

9. *Answer:* B
   Rationale: Responses A, C, and D are appropriate interventions to reduce hair loss. Heated rollers, a permanent, and hair coloring may actually speed hair loss.

10. *Answer:* B
    Rationale: Regrowth is rare before 1 month and after 6 months.

11. *Answer:* B
    Rationale: Chemotherapy drugs may affect all hair bulbs. Administration of multiple drugs may increase the severity of hair loss. Hair loss is usually not permanent with chemotherapy but may be permanent with radiation treatment.

12. *Answer:* C
    Rationale: Hair loss is the most common side effect listed. The other responses are not side effects of paclitaxel (Taxol).

13. *Answer:* B
    Rationale: Chemotherapy generally causes temporary hair loss. Radiation doses above 4500 cGy generally induce permanent loss.

14. *Answer:* C
    Rationale: Responses A, B, and D contain incorrect information (loss generally is faster with high doses of drugs with high potential for alopecia). Permanent and color may damage hair, thus increasing hair loss.

BIBLIOGRAPHY

Bello, L.K., & McIntire, S.N. (1995). Body image disturbances in young adults with cancer. *Cancer Nurs 18*(2), 138–143.

Ellis, J. (1991). How adolescents cope with cancer and its treatment. *MCN 16*(3), 157–160.

Freedman, T.G. (1994). Social and cultural dimensions of

hair loss in women treated for breast cancer. *Cancer Nurs 17*(4), 334–341.

Hopwood, P. (1993). The assessment of body image in cancer patients. *Eur J Cancer 29A*(2), 276–281.

Mock, V. (1993). Body image in women treated for breast cancer. *Nurs Res 42*(3), 153–157.

Pickard-Holley, S. (1995). The symptom experience of alopecia. *Semin Oncol Nurs 11*(4), 235–238.

Price, B. (1992). Living with altered body image: The cancer experience. *Br J Nurs 1*(13), 641–645.

NOTES

4

Cultural Issues

Joanne K. Itano

Select the best answer for each of the following questions:

1. Which of the following groups has the highest incidence of cancer for all sites combined?
   A. Caucasian males.
   B. African American males.
   C. Native American females.
   D. Native Hawaiian females.

2. African American males have the highest incidence of which of the following cancer(s)?
   A. Colon and rectum.
   B. Breast.
   C. Prostate.
   D. Liver.

3. Which of the following ethnic groups has the lowest incidence of cancer?
   A. Alaskan Natives.
   B. Native Americans.
   C. Hispanic Americans.
   D. Chinese Americans.

4. Women of which ethnic group have the highest mortality rate for invasive breast cancer?
   A. Native Hawaiian.
   B. Chinese American.
   C. Hispanic American.
   D. African American.

5. When caring for culturally diverse clients, the nurse needs to be concerned about avoiding ethnocentricity. Likely sources of ethnocentricity for the nurse include
   A. the health care system.
   B. the client's ethnicity.

C. the family's view of the illness.
D. all of the above.

6. A 72-year-old Native American woman with advanced cancer is comatose. She has a small discolored pouch around her neck. While bathing her, the most appropriate action for the nurse is to
   A. discard the pouch as it is a source of infection.
   B. remove it and place it in the drawer as you would any personal belongings.
   C. leave it on.
   D. remove it and talk with the family when they come.

7. The nurse would be most cautious when entering the personal space of which of the following clients?
   A. A 52-year-old African American woman.
   B. A 36-year-old Native American man.
   C. A 62-year-old Vietnamese man.
   D. A 40-year-old Hispanic woman.

8. Suggesting whole milk or cheese as a means to improve nutritional status should be used with caution for which of the following ethnic groups?
   A. Asian Americans and African Americans.
   B. Hispanic Americans.
   C. Native Americans and American Eskimos.
   D. Native Hawaiians.

9. A major factor explaining the differences in cancer incidence, mortality, and survival within different ethnic groups is
   A. skin color.
   B. generation immigrated to United States.

C. language.
D. poverty.

10. A wife has been at her husband's bedside continually since his admission 3 days ago. She is clearly tired. In considering their Japanese American background, the most appropriate nursing action is to
    A. insist that the wife go home at night.
    B. talk with the client to have him tell his wife to go home at night.
    C. do nothing as it is the wife's duty to be at the bedside at all times.

    D. talk with the family about other family members who might help stay with the client.

11. In assessing a client's beliefs about the cause of his cancer, he states that it is caused by an imbalance in nature. This is an example of which health belief system?
    A. Magico-religious.
    B. Biomedical.
    C. Holistic health.
    D. Fatalistic.

NOTES

ANSWERS

1. *Answer:* B
   Rationale: According to SEER incidence rates, 1988–1992, African American males have the highest incidence rates for all sites combined at 560/100,000 population.

2. *Answer:* C
   Rationale: According to SEER incidence rates, 1988–1992, African American males have the highest incidence of cancers of the esophagus, kidney/kidney pelvis, larynx, lung, multiple myeloma, oral cavity (excluding nasopharynx), pancreas, and prostate.

3. *Answer:* B
   Rationale: The 1988–1992 SEER data indicate that the incidence rate for Native Americans is 196/100,000 for males and 99/100,000 for females compared with white males at 469 and white females at 346. Although Native Americans have the lowest cancer incidence rates and rank mid to low in cancer mortality rates, these rates may reflect their shorter life span rather than a true lower incidence and mortality rate. Native Americans also have the lowest 5-year relative survival rates among the ethnic groups.

4. *Answer:* D
   Rationale: According to SEER mortality data, 1988–1992, the mortality rate from invasive breast cancer is 31.4/100,000 for African Americans, followed by Native Hawaiians with a rate of 25/100,000 and Caucasian women at 27/100,000.

5. *Answer:* A
   Rationale: Ethnocentrism is the tendency to view people unconsciously by using one's group and one's own customs as the standard for all judgments. Thus the sources of ethnocentrism for the nurse would be her or his own ethnicity and cultural beliefs and beliefs of the health care system of which she or he is a part.

6. *Answer:* C
   Rationale: Native Americans may carry objects believed to guard against witchcraft or have objects that are considered curative, given to the client by the native healers. The latter may be considered sacred. As long as the object does not interfere with the client's care, there is no harm to leaving it on. If for some reason it needs to be removed, consult with the family first since the client is comatose.

7. *Answer:* C
   Rationale: In general Asians are noncontact people compared with the other ethnic groups. They may feel uncomfortable with close physical contact.

8. *Answer:* A
   Rationale: Lactose intolerance is high in both of these groups.

9. *Answer:* D
   Rationale: Poverty, not race, accounts for a 10% to 15% lower survival rate from cancer in many ethnic groups. One researcher found that when data are corrected for economic status, African Americans had a slightly lower incidence and mortality for a number of cancers than did Caucasian Americans. The disproportionate number of African Americans in the lower socioeconomic strata accounted for the increased incidence. In another study when only Caucasians who received the same level of care were included in the study, it was found that indigent clients regardless of ethnicity had poorer survival rates for each cancer type. The impact of poverty on cancer is felt in ethnic minorities since a disproportionate number of ethnic minorities comprise the poor of America.

10. *Answer:* D
    Rationale: There is an expectation for the wife to be the primary caretaker in the Japanese culture. Other family members may also share the duties. To "not bother the nurses" is also a common belief. Choices A and B do not consider their cultural beliefs, whereas choice C does. However, it does not consider the health of the wife and possible caregiver burnout.

11. *Answer:* C
    Rationale: In this health belief view the forces of nature must be in balance or in harmony. Human life is one aspect of nature and must be in harmony with the rest of nature. Native Americans often have this view. Health and illness are controlled by supernatural forces is the

belief in the magico-religious view. Some African Americans may believe in voodoo, whereas Hispanic Americans often believe that illness is caused by the evil eye (mal ojo). The biomedical health belief view is that life and life processes are controlled by physical and biochemical processes that can be manipulated by humans. The client will expect medications, a treatment, or surgery to cure the health problem.

BIBLIOGRAPHY

Barkauskas, V., Stoltenberg-Allen, K., Baumann, L., et al. (1994). Cultural considerations in health assessment. In V. Baukauskas, K. Stoltenberg-Allen, L.C. Baumann, & C. Darling-Fisher (eds.). *Health and Physical Assessment.* St. Louis: Mosby–Year Book, pp. 149–181.

Frank-Stromborg, M., & Olsen, S.J. (eds.). (1993). *Cancer Prevention in Minority Populations: Cultural Implications for Health Care Professionals.* St. Louis: Mosby–Year Book.

Giger, J.N., & Davidhizar, R.E. (1995). *Transcultural Nursing: Assessment and Intervention.* St. Louis: Mosby.

Itano, J. (1998). Cultural issues. In J. Itano & K. Taoka (eds.). *Core Curriculum in Oncology Nursing* (3rd ed.). Philadelphia: WB Saunders, pp. 60–76.

Kagawa-Singer, M. (1996). Cultural systems. In R. McCorkle, M. Grant, M.J. Frank-Stromborg, & S. Baird (eds.). *Cancer Nursing: A Comprehensive Textbook* (2nd ed.). Philadelphia: WB Saunders, pp. 38–52.

Lipson, J.G., Dibble, S.L., & Minarik, P.A. (eds.). (1996). *Culture and Nursing Care: A Pocket Guide.* San Francisco: UCSF Nursing Press.

Spector, R. (1996). *Cultural Diversity in Health and Illness* (4th ed.). Stamford, CT: Appleton & Lange.

Taoka, K., & Itano, J. (1997). Cultural diversity among individuals with cancer. In S. Groenwald, M. Goodman, M. Frogge, & C. Yarbro (eds.). *Cancer Nursing: Principles and Practice* (4th ed.). Boston: Jones & Barlett, pp. 1691–1735.

Wilkes, G., Freeman, H., & Prout, M. (1994). Cancer and poverty: Breaking the cycle. *Semin Oncol Nurs 10,* 79–88.

NOTES

5

Coping: Survivorship Issues and Financial Concerns

Susan Leigh

Select the best answer for each of the following questions:

1. Approximately 51% of the 7.4 million Americans with histories of cancer have survived longer than 5 years. How many are considered cancer survivors according to consumer groups such as the National Coalition for Cancer Survivorship (NCCS)?
   A. About 5 million.
   B. All 7.4 million.
   C. Anyone who has completed treatment.
   D. Anyone who has not had a recurrence of disease.

2. Survivorship in relation to cancer is a relatively new concept. Initially described by NCCS, survivorship encompasses all the following concepts *except*
   A. survivorship proceeds along a continuum through and beyond treatment to remissions, recurrences, cure, and the final stages of life.
   B. survivorship is a dynamic, evolutionary process.
   C. survivorship is a predetermined stage of survival that begins 5 years after treatment ends and only describes clients who are cured.
   D. survivorship issues also affect family members, significant others, friends, coworkers, health care professionals, and social support networks.

3. Which stage of survival includes the initial diagnosis and treatment?
   A. The extended or intermediate stage.
   B. The permanent or long-term stage.
   C. The terminal stage.
   D. The acute or immediate stage.

4. During the acute or immediate stage of survival, survivors would *rarely* encounter
   A. the fear of dying.
   B. acute side effects from therapy.
   C. late or delayed effects of treatment.
   D. disruption in family and social roles.

5. Survivors in the extended or intermediate stage of survival are
   A. finished completely with all medical treatments.
   B. in remission or receiving maintenance therapy.
   C. considered "cured" of their disease.
   D. undergoing initial therapy.

6. Which statement *best* characterizes a survivor in the permanent or long-term stage of survival?
   A. The survivor's cancer status has gradually evolved to where the probability for disease recurrence is minimal.
   B. The survivor is cancer free.
   C. The survivor is guaranteed to be cured.
   D. The survivor has reached the 5-year disease-free mark after completing therapy.

7. Which of the following *best* describes symptoms or effects that persist for months or years after therapy has been completed?
    A. Progressive effects.
    B. Iatrogenic effects.
    C. Erroneous effects.
    D. Long-term effects.

8. Examples of late or delayed effects of cancer therapy include all of the following *except*
    A. second malignancies.
    B. radiation erythema.
    C. pulmonary fibrosis.
    D. cardiomyopathy.

9. A 32-year-old woman who had been treated for Hodgkin's disease at the age of 17 now has breast cancer. Which of the following statements does *not* necessarily apply to second malignancies?
    A. It is possible that this second malignancy was a result of prior mantle radiation therapy.
    B. The overall risk of second malignancies is relatively low but remains a serious problem for those affected.
    C. The risk of second malignancies does not contraindicate therapy for the first malignancy.
    D. No therapy should ever be given if it creates a risk for other malignancies.

10. All of the following statements are false *except*
    A. most cancer survivors have severe and permanent psychological impairment.
    B. after therapy is completed, there is no need for continued psychosocial support.
    C. the fear of recurrence may persist for many years, and possibly forever, after completion of therapy.
    D. the Damocles syndrome refers to a genetic predisposition to cancer.

11. Although employment discrimination continues to haunt survivors, there are laws that offer protection to people with histories of cancer. When survivors qualify for new jobs, promotions, or retention of existing jobs, current laws
    A. are the same laws that protect the mentally or physically disabled.
    B. are only legislated through state governments.
    C. only apply to private employers.
    D. have a statute of limitations.

12. Which one of the following statements about health insurance is *not* true?
    A. Portability of insurance and deletion of the preexisting conditions clause from insurance will be modest improvements in insuring people with histories of cancer.
    B. Insurance companies may reduce existing benefits of a policy after a cancer diagnosis.
    C. New applications for insurance can never be legally refused.
    D. Insurance policies for survivors cost more and take longer to obtain.

13. Many survivors critically examine their lives and search for meaning after a cancer experience. How well they live can become as important as how long they live, and many survivors experience an increased appreciation and zest for life. This describes
    A. spiritual or existential issues that are affected by a cancer experience and that are individual and personal.
    B. emotional trauma that lingers indefinitely after cancer.
    C. psychological issues that warrant therapy.
    D. none of the above.

14. Survivor's guilt can be described as
    A. a spiritual or existential issue.
    B. a phenomenon experienced during routine follow-up visits when confronted with others who are not doing well, are more debilitated, or are terminal.
    C. a normal reaction to surviving a life-threatening experience.
    D. all of the above.

15. Ideally, long-term follow-up care for cancer survivors would include
    A. education on prevention, early detection, and health promotion.
    B. assessment of all prior therapies and risk factors.
    C. psychosocial interview and referrals as necessary.
    D. all of the above.

ANSWERS

1. *Answer:* B
Rationale: According to the NCCS and many cancer survivors themselves, the survival journey begins at the moment of diagnosis: *"from the time of its discovery and for the balance of life, an individual diagnosed with cancer is a survivor."*

2. *Answer:* C
Rationale: Rather than a predetermined time frame, survivorship can be viewed as living with, through, or beyond a diagnosis of cancer, regardless of outcome, and affects both those with the diagnosis and others who care about and for them.

3. *Answer:* D
Rationale: The acute or immediate stage of survival signifies the beginning of the cancer experience when the client undergoes a diagnostic work-up followed by therapy.

4. *Answer:* C
Rationale: Late or delayed effects of treatment usually occur months to years after therapy is completed.

5. *Answer:* B
Rationale: When disease is in remission or survivors have completed the basic, rigorous course of treatment, the extended or intermediate stage has begun. They may or may not continue to receive maintenance therapy and will not know for years whether treatment has been successful.

6. *Answer:* A
Rationale: This stage is roughly equated with "cure," yet there is no such thing as a guarantee. Rather than a guarantee of cure, there is a gradual evolution from the extended stage of survival into a period where the likelihood of disease recurrence is sufficiently small that the cancer can be considered permanently arrested.

7. *Answer:* D
Rationale: Long-term effects of cancer and cancer therapy begin during the acute or extended stages and continue indefinitely after treatment ends. Many of these effects gradually subside (e.g., hair regrows), whereas others can become chronic conditions (e.g., neuropathies).

8. *Answer:* B
Rationale: Unlike erythema, late effects are clinically obvious, clinically subtle, or subclinical sequelae that may become apparent months to years after completion of treatment.

9. *Answer:* D
Rationale: The chance for survival and potential cure would not be possible without current therapies. The risk/benefit ratio for specific treatment options must be weighed; survivors must be aware of these risks; and continued medical surveillance must be lifelong.

10. *Answer:* C
Rationale: Although much of the fear associated with cancer gradually subsides after treatment is completed, an underlying fear of recurrence, sometimes called the Damocles syndrome, can remain with survivors forever. This fear can be triggered at the time of medical follow-up visits, during an anniversary of diagnosis or treatment completion, or at any time a suspicious symptom arises. Although survivors have varying needs for continued psychosocial support after therapy, few are considered to have overt mental illness because of their cancer diagnosis.

11. *Answer:* A
Rationale: In general, denial of employment solely because of a cancer history to cancer survivors who are qualified for the jobs violates most laws that prohibit discrimination against the handicapped. Cancer survivors are protected under the premise that they are *perceived* to be handicapped as opposed to having outright disabilities. For these laws to be effective, though, they must be tested in state or federal courts of law or in both.

12. *Answer:* C
Rationale: Adequate health insurance is rarely guaranteed and continues to be a major obstacle to social recovery for many cancer survivors. The problems created when a survivor attempts to secure or obtain these benefits can be financially and emotionally devastating. Even

with new legislation that supposedly guarantees portability and eliminates the preexisting conditions clause, there is no limit on how much the insurance industry can charge for coverage.

13. *Answer:* A

Rationale: Surviving a life-threatening experience often heightens the desire to get on with living and personally evaluate life's priorities and meaning. Some survivors become more religious. Others feel a deepened sense of spirituality. Few survivors can deny a certain sense of transformation.

14. *Answer:* D

Rationale: Comparisons may be made with other clients, causing survivors to wonder, Why am I doing well and they aren't? Similar to questions arising around the time of initial diagnosis, attempts to justify "why me" or "why not me" may resurface. Hence the survivor's ongoing involvement with follow-up care is characterized by mixed emotional reactions and multiple concerns and is a normal part of the overall situation.

15. *Answer:* D

Rationale: Follow-up for cancer survivors is a lifelong responsibility and needs to include strategies to enhance the early detection of recurrent disease and to reduce the risk for second malignancies. Also, new behaviors to enhance overall wellness should be promoted. Examples of interventions include sessions on nutrition, exercise, smoking cessation, stress reduction, group support, and individual therapy.

BIBLIOGRAPHY

Ferrell, B.R., Hassey Dow, K., Leigh, S., Ly, J., & Gulasefaram, P. (1995). Quality of life in long-term cancer survivors. *Oncol Nurs Forum 22*(6), 915–922.

Hoffman, B. (1996). *A Cancer Survivor's Almanac: Charting Your Journey.* Minneapolis: Chronimed Publishing.

Leigh, S., Welch-McCaffrey, D., Loescher, L.J., & Hoffman, B. (1993). Psychosocial issues of long-term survival from adult cancer. In S.L. Groenwald, M.H. Frogge, M. Goodman, & C.H. Yarbro (eds.). *Cancer Nursing: Principles and Practice* (3rd ed.). Boston: Jones & Bartlett, pp. 484–495.

Leigh, S. (1998). Coping: Survivorship issues and financial concerns. In J. Itano & K. Taoka (eds.). *Core Curriculum for Oncology Nursing* (3rd ed.). Philadelphia: WB Saunders.

Schwartz, C.L., Hobbie, W.L., Constine, L.S., & Ruccione, K.S. (1994). *Survivors of Childhood Cancer: Assessment and Management.* St. Louis: Mosby.

NOTES

6

Sexuality

Patricia W. Nishimoto

Select the best answer for each of the following questions:

1. A special focus on issues of sexuality is warranted where clients are
   A. single.
   B. terminally ill.
   C. elderly.
   D. newly diagnosed.

2. The PLISSIT (Permission, Limited Information, Specific Suggestions, Intensive Therapy) model for sexuality counseling
   A. can only be used by nurses with an advanced degree.
   B. does not require any knowledge about sexuality or how sexuality is affected by a diagnosis of cancer or the treatment for cancer.
   C. is a useful model for levels of nursing interventions based on the nurse's comfort and knowledge about the subject.
   D. is used primarily for clients with long-standing or severe problems with sexuality.

3. If a pregnant woman is diagnosed with cancer,
   A. she should be counseled about the need for an immediate therapeutic termination of pregnancy.
   B. her prognosis will be much worse since pregnancy increases the rate of growth of the malignancy.
   C. diagnosis at an earlier stage of disease will be easier than for a woman who was not pregnant.

   D. she will need high-risk obstetric care and to have her diagnostic work-up and treatment plan evaluated for risk to the fetus and herself.

4. If a woman decides to receive treatment while she is pregnant,
   A. the choice of chemotherapy will not be an issue.
   B. high-risk prenatal care will be necessary because of the risk of thrombocytopenia, disseminated intravascular coagulation, and premature delivery.
   C. only chemotherapy and radiation therapy will be risks to the fetus.
   D. she will need to be referred for psychiatric evaluation for potential fetal abuse.

5. Sexual dysfunction as a result of radiation therapy is
   A. dependent on the source of radiation and the area of the radiation field.
   B. usually psychologic, because radiation therapy poses few physiologic threats to sexual functioning.
   C. rare in women.
   D. is easily corrected with the use of antidepressants.

6. What physiologic changes *do not* occur in women having external pelvic irradiation?
   A. Decreased vaginal lubrication.
   B. Radioactivity of the vagina.
   C. Shortening of the vaginal vault.
   D. Decreased elasticity of the vagina.

7. Sexual dysfunction secondary to chemo-therapy
    A. results primarily from damage to the penis or the vagina.
    B. is of little concern to "normal patients" but may be of importance to clients with a psychiatric history.
    C. indicates treatment should be discontinued.
    D. needs to be assessed since sexuality issues can directly affect quality of life.

8. Which of the following is a *true* statement about fertility after chemotherapy?
    A. The age of a client when treated will not affect future fertility.
    B. The type of chemotherapy is not a significant factor when future fertility is a consideration.
    C. Administration of a single drug versus combination chemotherapy may affect future fertility.
    D. Low sperm counts at 1 year after treatment completion indicate a permanent condition.

9. Which of the following psychological responses to treatment or disease can affect sexual functioning?
    A. Anxiety.
    B. Feeling of isolation.
    C. Heightened sense of vulnerability.
    D. All of the above.

10. Which side effect is *not* caused by hormonal therapy?
    A. Gynecomastia.
    B. Erectile dysfunction.
    C. Penile or testicular atrophy.
    D. Priapism.

11. Which surgical intervention does *not* affect sexual functioning/sexuality?
    A. Prostatectomy.
    B. Radical abdominal lymph node dissection.
    C. Unilateral orchiectomy.
    D. Head and neck surgery.

12. Education and anticipatory guidance to prevent sexual dysfunction include
    A. assuming the client knows basic sexuality information.
    B. encouraging the couple to avoid discussing fears or concerns with each other.
    C. dispelling myths or misconceptions.
    D. using models or drawings to explain how sexuality can be affected.

13. Which is *not* a desired client outcome of nursing interventions to improve sexuality?
    A. Identifies potential or actual alterations in sexuality related to disease or treatment.
    B. Identifies satisfactory alternative methods for expressing sexuality that is consistent with client values and culture.
    C. Identifies strategies to break up relationships to protect the partner from the need to cope with terminal illness.
    D. Identifies personal and community resources to assist with changes in body image and sexuality.

14. As a nurse caring for Mr. C. after an abdominoperineal resection, which of the following client or significant other concerns are most realistic to discuss with him?
    A. Awareness of a variety of ways for sexual pleasure.
    B. Ability to ejaculate with intercourse.
    C. Security in his masculinity after surgery.
    D. Ability to achieve an erection after surgery.

15. Mrs. J. is scheduled to have a mastectomy for breast cancer. Which of the following questions would be *most* appropriate for the nurse to ask when discussing the potential impact of surgery on sexuality?
    A. Do you have any concerns about how the loss of your breast may affect how others see you?
    B. Some women have concerns about the effects the surgery will have on their sexual life. Do you have any concerns?
    C. Do you have any problems with your sexual life at this time?
    D. Some women don't see themselves as feminine after the surgery. Do you?

16. Mrs. G. has been told to use a vaginal dilator after radiation therapy to the cervix. Which of

the following statements is the most appropriate for the nurse to use in teaching Mrs. G.?

A. Insert the dilator into your vagina as quickly as possible.
B. Lubricate the dilator with an oil-based jelly.
C. Leave the dilator inserted for 10 minutes each time.
D. Wait 6 weeks after radiation to begin using the dilator.

17. Mrs. T. is receiving radiation therapy to the pelvis. She states that she has not had intercourse for several weeks, although she desires sexual intimacy. Which of the following suggestions would be most appropriate for the nurse to make to Mrs. T.?

A. Let your partner know you are interested in having sex.
B. Limit the amount of time you and your partner initially spend on intercourse.
C. Ask your partner why he hasn't wanted to have sex.
D. Concentrate on pleasing your partner during intercourse.

NOTES

ANSWERS

1. *Answer:* D
   Rationale: The issue of sexuality needs to be addressed for each client, regardless of marital status, age, culture, and so on. The nurse needs to incorporate those factors into the assessment but not use them as factors for decisions of whether to speak to the client about sexuality.

2. *Answer:* C
   Rationale: This model allows health care providers to obtain the information to plan interventions at the appropriate level based on their ability and identified client needs.

3. *Answer:* D
   Rationale: The issue of termination would depend on the type of disease, doubling time of the malignancy, and the gestational age of the fetus. Diagnostic work-ups can be adjusted to reduce the amount of risk to the fetus. Different chemotherapy agents can be given during specific trimesters. Radiation therapy may be delayed until after delivery.

4. *Answer:* B
   Rationale: Surgery, hormonal therapy, immunotherapy, and diagnostic tests may be a risk to the fetus. A decision not to abort but to have treatment while pregnant is not "fetal abuse."

5. *Answer:* A
   Rationale: Pelvic irradiation may decrease vaginal lubrication and elasticity of the vagina and shorten the vaginal vault. Sexual dysfunction after radiation therapy may have both psychologic and physiologic bases.

6. *Answer:* B
   Rationale: External radiation therapy does not cause a body part to be "radioactive" and a danger to others. This may be a fear or concern of the client or her partner, thus creating sexual dysfunction, but it is not a physiologic change.

7. *Answer:* D
   Rationale: Sexual dysfunction resulting from chemotherapy is usually temporary and can be related to nausea, fatigue, decreased vaginal lubrication, body image changes from alopecia, and so on.

8. *Answer:* C
   Rationale: Fertility is affected in 80% of men who receive MOPP. Effects on fertility from many drugs are reversible. This may be reversed as late as 4 years after treatment.

9. *Answer:* D
   Rationale: Anxiety, feelings of isolation, and a heightened sense of vulnerability can all affect sexual functioning.

10. *Answer:* D
    Rationale: This is not a hormone-related condition.

11. *Answer:* C
    Rationale: Unilateral orchiectomy preserves some hormone production. Nerve damage during prostatectomy may cause retrograde ejaculation or erectile dysfunction. Head and neck surgery changes in appearance and ability to speak may affect self-image or the partner's sexual desire but not function per se.

12. *Answer:* C
    Rationale: Myths or misconceptions can escalate anxiety and interfere with sexual functioning.

13. *Answer:* C
    Rationale: All of the other responses are appropriate. C assumes that any person with a diagnosis of cancer is terminally ill. It also incorrectly assumes that a partner will not grieve if he or she separates from the client before the client dies.

14. *Answer:* A
    Rationale: With an abdominoperineal resection, the client most likely will not be able to sustain an erection and will have retrograde ejaculation. The client most likely will not internalize the effect of these changes on his self-concept before leaving the hospital.

15. *Answer:* B
    Rationale: The correct answer provides permission for sexual concerns. By using "some

women . . ." an opportunity is provided for the client to express her individual concerns.

16. *Answer:* C

Rationale: The vaginal dilator is used to maintain the vaginal space and minimize the stenotic effects of radiation therapy. However, the effectiveness of intervention depends on the correct technique and consistency of use.

17. *Answer:* A

Rationale: Often the partner is reluctant to initiate sexual activities for fear of hurting the client or because the partner assumes that the client does not want to have sex.

BIBLIOGRAPHY

Cartwright-Alzarese, F. (1995). Addressing sexual dysfunction following radiation therapy for a gynecologic malignancy. *Oncol Nurs Forum 22*(8), 1227–1232.

Ghizzani, A., Pirtolli, L., & Bellazza, A. (1995). The evaluation of some factors influencing the sexual life of women affected by breast cancer. *J Sex Marital Ther 21*(1), 57–63.

Hughes, M.K. (1996). Sexuality changes in the cancer patient. *Nurs Interventions Oncol 8,* 15.

Lamb, M.A. (1995). Effects of cancer on the sexuality and fertility of women. *Semin Oncol Nurs 11*(2), 120–127.

Nishimoto, P.W. (1995). Sex and sexuality in the cancer patient. *Nurs Pract Forum 6*(4), 221–227.

Nishimoto, P.W. (1998). Sexuality. In J.K. Itano & K.N. Taoka (eds.). *Core Curriculum for Oncology Nursing* (3rd ed.). Philadelphia: WB Saunders, pp. 85–95.

NOTES

7

Symptom Management and Supportive Care: Dying and Death

June Lunney

Select the best answer for each of the following questions:

1. Which of the following is the *best* example of an ethical dilemma?
   - A. Use of heavy sedation to manage refractory pain.
   - B. Family decision to withhold hydration from a comatose dying client.
   - C. Son's insistence on kidney dialysis for his mother in spite of her objections.
   - D. Refusal of chemotherapy by a lung cancer client with brain metastasis.

2. Mr. T. has just begun a titration dose of morphine for severe pain. You may expect to see all of the following *except*
   - A. mental clouding.
   - B. constipation.
   - C. urinary retention.
   - D. rapid respirations.

3. Which type of pain is caused by bone metastasis?
   - A. Nociceptive.
   - B. Visceral.
   - C. Neuropathic.
   - D. Complex regional pain syndromes.

4. Mrs. R., who is terminally ill, reports feeling nauseated. Your first response should be to
   - A. suggest dietary changes.
   - B. teach her family to use antiemetics.
   - C. teach distraction and relaxation techniques.
   - D. assess for constipation.

5. You find Mr. K. gasping and panting. He tells you that he is petrified of suffocating to death. Which of the following is an incorrect response to the situation?
   - A. Temporarily withholding opioids.
   - B. Auscultating breath sounds in all fields.
   - C. Repositioning him in a sitting position.
   - D. Teaching relaxation techniques.

6. Perceptual disturbances, clouded consciousness, delusions, hallucinations, and sleep disturbances are most characteristic of
   - A. dementia.
   - B. anxiety disorder.
   - C. delirium.
   - D. selective cognitive impairment.

7. Which of the following is *not* true about dehydration in the terminally ill?
   - A. Dehydration is predictable and does not necessarily warrant an attempt to reverse the condition.
   - B. A major physical problem associated with dehydration is dry mouth.
   - C. Dehydration is an emotional issue for the family.
   - D. A major negative effect of dehydration is decreased urine output.

8. Mr. J. is experiencing insomnia, fatigue, anorexia, and a diminished ability to concentrate. Your most appropriate response would be to
   A. talk with him about his fears of dying.
   B. encourage family members to spend more time with him.
   C. further evaluate him for depression.
   D. reduce his next dose of opioids.

9. Mr. F., who is dying, finds it difficult to eat. Your appropriate response is to
   A. encourage his wife to make small portions of his favorite foods.
   B. request that his physician consider prescribing megestrol.
   C. explain the multiple causes of anorexia to his family.
   D. recommend a course of total parenteral nutrition.

10. Appropriate interventions to facilitate family coping with advanced illness include all of the following *except*
   A. recognizing areas of concurrent stress not related to the client's illness.
   B. providing opportunities for caregivers to express negative emotions.
   C. discouraging conflict among family members.
   D. developing family education about the basic physical aspects of caregiving.

11. The best example of a good problem-focused coping mechanism for nurses to deal with the stress of caring for terminally ill clients is
   A. expressing feelings of helplessness.
   B. increasing competency in pain assessment.
   C. attending an institutional support group.
   D. retreating from social interactions.

12. Mrs. S. has just died. In providing bereavement care, you appropriately would choose to do all of the following *except*
   A. express your sympathy to the family.
   B. provide information about bereavement services.
   C. ask about other death experiences in the family.
   D. delay contacting the family until at least 8 weeks after the death.

13. Mrs. E. reports that she has not had a bowel movement in 6 days. She is of the Muslim faith. Which of the following will most likely affect your care for her?
   A. Fatalism.
   B. Modesty.
   C. Islamic ritual.
   D. Observance of Ramadan.

14. Lucy O. is an 11-year-old dying of leukemia. You should be most concerned about
   A. her possible physical dependence on analgesia.
   B. her not understanding that she is dying.
   C. the death images in her art work.
   D. headache pain.

15. Hospice care is not appropriate for the following:
   A. Clients who are responding to treatment.
   B. Clients who wish to receive artificial hydration.
   C. Clients who are maintaining an active social life.
   D. Clients who need intensive pain management.

ANSWERS

1. *Answer:* C
Rationale: Client autonomy in clinical decision making is a high priority. However, metabolic consequences associated with the need for dialysis can affect an individual's capacity to think clearly.

2. *Answer:* D
Rationale: Initiation of morphine may lead to depressed or slowed respiration.

3. *Answer:* A
Rationale: Somatic or nociceptive pain occurs as a result of activation of deep musculoskeletal tissues.

4. *Answer:* D
Rationale: Constipation may cause nausea. Corrective measures to eliminate the cause of nausea and vomiting are the appropriate first steps to take.

5. *Answer:* A
Rationale: Opioids can reduce breathlessness, which would be appropriate in this case.

6. *Answer:* C
Rationale: Delirium is a reversible organic mental disorder with general cognitive impairment. Dementia is not associated with clouded consciousness but with a normally alert state.

7. *Answer:* D
Rationale: Although decreased urine output is an effect of dehydration, with a dying client it is a positive effect because of the associated decrease in incontinence.

8. *Answer:* C
Rationale: Insomnia, fatigue, anorexia, and a diminished ability to concentrate are symptoms of depression. Antidepressants are appropriate for dying clients.

9. *Answer:* C
Rationale: Explaining the multiple causes of anorexia to the family helps them to accept the loss of appetite. Encouraging the client with favorite foods may induce guilt on the part of the client and family.

10. *Answer:* C
Rationale: It is a better option to allow the family members to express and resolve conflict than to discourage such discussion.

11. *Answer:* B
Rationale: Increasing competence is a problem-focused approach to stress management. Expressing concerns is an emotion-based approach.

12. *Answer:* D
Rationale: Between 3 and 8 weeks after the death the family members are often on their own and grief is at its peak.

13. *Answer:* B
Rationale: A woman of the Muslim faith is likely to be so modest that she is not able to manage allowing another person to check for a fecal impaction.

14. *Answer:* D
Rationale: Leukemias can cause meningeal irritation and obstruction with increased intracranial pressure.

15. *Answer:* A
Rationale: Hospice care cannot appropriately treat clients who are actively seeking to cure their illness.

BIBLIOGRAPHY

Barale, K. (1991). Nutritional support. In S.B. Baird, M.G. Donehower, V. Stalsbroten, & T.B. Ades (eds.). *A Cancer Source Book for Nurses* (6th ed.). Atlanta: The American Cancer Society.

Benner, P. (1991). Stress and coping with cancer. In S.B. Baird, R. McCorkle, & M. Grant (eds.). *Cancer Nursing: A Comprehensive Textbook.* Philadelphia: WB Saunders, pp. 717–741.

Burns, N., & Holmes, B.C. (1991). Alterations in body image. In S.B. Baird, R. McCorkle, & M. Grant (eds.). *Cancer Nursing: A Comprehensive Textbook.* Philadelphia: WB Saunders, pp. 821–830.

Carnevali, D.L., & Reiner, A.C. (1990). *The Cancer Experience: Nursing Diagnosis and Management.* Philadelphia: JB Lippincott.

Carpenito, L.J. (1983). *Nursing Diagnosis: Application to Clinical Practice.* Philadelphia: JB Lippincott.

Chamorro, T. (1991). Cancer and sexuality. In S.B. Baird, M.G. Donehower, V. Stalsbroten, & T.B. Ades (eds.). *A*

Cancer Source Book for Nurses (6th ed.). Atlanta: The American Cancer Society, pp. 141–149.

Clark, J.C. (1990). Psychosocial dimensions: The patient. In S.L. Groenwald, M.H. Frogge, M. Goodman, & C.H. Yarbro (eds.). *Cancer Nursing: Principles and Practice* (2nd ed.). Boston: Jones & Bartlett Publishers, pp. 346–364.

Cooper, C.L. (ed.). (1984). *Psychosocial Stress and Cancer.* New York: John Wiley & Sons.

Coyle, N., & Foley, K.M. (1991). Alterations in comfort: Pain. In S.B. Baird, R. McCorkle, & M. Grant (eds.). *Cancer Nursing: A Comprehensive Textbook.* Philadelphia: WB Saunders, pp. 782–805.

Donehower, M.G. (1991). Symptom management. In S.B. Baird, M.G. Donehower, V. Stalsbroten, & T.B. Ades (eds.). *A Cancer Source Book for Nurses* (6th ed.). Atlanta: The American Cancer Society, pp. 100–110.

Donoghue, M., Nunnally, C., & Yasko, J.M. (1982). *Nutritional Aspects of Cancer Care.* Reston, VA: Reston Publishing.

Dudas, S. (1990). Altered body image and sexuality. In S.L. Groenwald, M.H. Frogge, M. Goodman, & C.H. Yarbro (eds.). *Cancer Nursing: Principles and Practice* (2nd ed.). Boston: Jones & Bartlett Publishers, pp. 581–593.

Fanslow, J. (1991). Pain management. In S.B. Baird, M.G. Donehower, V. Stalsbroten, & T.B. Ades (eds.). *A Cancer Source Book for Nurses* (6th ed.). Atlanta: The American Cancer Society, pp. 111–120.

Ferszt, G., & Barg, F.K. (1991). Psychosocial support. In S.B. Baird, M.G. Donehower, V. Stalsbroten, & T.B. Ades (eds.). *A Cancer Source Book for Nurses* (6th ed.). Atlanta: The American Cancer Society, pp. 150–158.

Gobel, B.H. (1990). Bleeding. In S.L. Groenwald, M.H. Frogge, M. Goodman, & C.H. Yarbro (eds.). *Cancer Nursing: Principles and Practice* (2nd ed.). Boston: Jones & Bartlett Publishers, pp. 467–484.

Griffiths, M.J., Murray, K.H., & Russo, P.C. (1984). *Oncology Nursing: Pathophysiology, Assessment, and Intervention.* New York: Macmillan Publishing.

Holland, J.C., & Massie, M.J. (1988). *Psychiatric Management of Anxiety in Patients With Cancer.* Chicago: Upjohn.

Hughes, J. (1986). Denial in cancer patients. In B.A. Stroll (ed.). *Coping With Cancer Stress.* Boston: Martinus Nijhoff Publishers, pp. 63–70.

Hughes, J. (1986). Depression in cancer patients. In B.A. Stroll (ed.). *Coping With Cancer Stress.* Boston: Martinus Nijhoff Publishers, pp. 53–62.

Jacobs, M.M., & Geels, W. (eds.). (1985). *Signs and Symptoms in Nursing: Interpretation and Management.* Philadelphia: JB Lippincott.

Jalowiec, A., & Dudas, S. (1991). Alterations in patient coping. In S.B. Baird, R. McCorkle, & M. Grant (eds.). *Cancer Nursing: A Comprehensive Textbook.* Philadelphia: WB Saunders, pp. 806–820.

Johnson, B.L., & Gross, J. (eds.). (1985). *Handbook of Oncology Nursing.* New York: John Wiley & Sons.

Kaye, P. (1989). *Notes on Symptom Control in Hospice and Palliative Care.* Essex, CT: Hospice Education Institute, pp. 139–146.

Klemm, P.R., & Hubbard, S.M. (1990). Infection. In S.L. Groenwald, M.H. Frogge, M. Goodman, & C.H. Yarbro (eds.). *Cancer Nursing: Principles and Practice* (2nd ed.). Boston: Jones & Bartlett Publishers, pp. 442–466.

Krebs, L.U. (1990). Sexual and reproductive dysfunction. In S.L. Groenwald, M.H. Frogge, M. Goodman, & C.H. Yarbro (eds.). *Cancer Nursing: Principles and Practice* (2nd ed.). Boston: Jones & Bartlett Publishers, pp. 563–580.

Lamb, M.A. (1991). Alteratins in sexuality and sexual functioning. In. S.B. Baird, R. McCorkle, & M. Grant (eds.). *Cancer Nursing: A Comprehensive Textbook.* Philadelphia: WB Saunders, pp. 821–830.

Lang-Kummer, J.M. (1990). Hypercalcemia. In S.L. Groenwald, M.H. Frogge, M. Goodman, & C.H. Yarbro (eds.). *Cancer Nursing: Principles and Practice* (2nd ed.). Boston: Jones & Bartlett Publishers, pp. 520–534.

Lydon, J., Purl, S., & Goodman, M. (1990). Integumentary and mucous membrane alterations. In S.L. Groenwald, M.H. Frogge, M. Goodman, & C.H. Yarbro (eds.). *Cancer Nursing: Principles and Practice* (2nd ed.). Boston: Jones & Bartlett Publishers, pp. 594–643.

McCaffery, M., & Beebe, A. (1989). *Pain: Clinical Manual for Nursing Practice.* St. Louis: C.V. Mosby.

McGee, R.F. (1990). Overview of psychosocial dimensions. In S.L. Groenwald, M.H. Frogge, M. Goodman, & C.H. Yarbro (eds.). *Cancer Nursing: Principles and Practice* (2nd ed.). Boston: Jones & Bartlett Publishers, pp. 341–345.

McGuire, D.B., & Sheidler, V.R. (1990). Pain. In S.L. Groenwald, M.H. Frogge, M. Goodman, & C.H. Yarbro (eds.). *Cancer Nursing: Principles and Practice* (2nd ed.). Boston: Jones & Bartlett Publishers, pp. 385–441.

McGuire, D.B., & Yarbro, C.H. (eds.). (1987). *Cancer Pain Management.* Orlando, FL: Grune & Stratton.

McNally, J.C., Somerville, E.T., Miaskowski, C., & Rostad, M. (eds.). (1991). *Guidelines for Oncology Nursing Practice* (2nd ed.). Philadelphia: WB Saunders.

Moore, L.M., & Ruccione, K. (1990). Late effects of cancer treatment. In S.L. Groenwald, M.H. Frogge, M. Goodman, & C.H. Yarbro (eds.). *Cancer Nursing: Principles and Practice* (2nd ed.). Boston: Jones & Bartlett Publishers, pp. 669–688.

Nail, L.M. (1990). Fatigue. In S.L. Groenwald, M.H. Frogge, M. Goodman, & C.H. Yarbro (eds.). *Cancer Nursing: Principles and Practice* (2nd ed.). Boston: Jones & Bartlett Publishers.

National Institute of Mental Health. (undated). *Depression: What You Need to Know.* Rockville, MD: U.S. Department of Health and Human Services.

North American Nursing Diagnosis Association. (1989). *Taxonomy 1 With Official Diagnosis Categories.* St. Louis: Author.

Piper, B.F. (1991). Alterations in energy: The sensation of fatigue. In S.B. Baird, R. McCorkle, & M. Grant (eds.). *Cancer Nursing: A Comprehensive Textbook.* Philadelphia: WB Saunders, pp. 894–908.

Snyder, M. (1985). *Independent Nursing Interventions.* New York: John Wiley & Sons.

Szeluga, D.J., Groenwald, S.L., & Sullivan, D.K. (1990). Nutritional disturbances. In S.L. Groenwald, M.H. Frogge, M. Goodman, & C.H. Yarbro (eds.). *Cancer Nursing: Principles and Practice* (2nd ed.). Boston: Jones & Bartlett Publishers, pp. 495–519.

Varricchio, C.G., Miller, N., & Pazdur, M. (1990). Edema and effusions. In S.L. Groenwald, M.H. Frogge, M. Goodman, & C.H. Yarbro (eds.). *Cancer Nursing: Principles and Practice* (2nd ed.). Boston: Jones & Bartlett Publishers, pp. 546–562.

Zerwekh, J. (1991). Supportive care for the dying patient. In S.B. Baird, R. McCorkle, & M. Grant (eds.). *Cancer Nursing: A Comprehensive Textbook.* Philadelphia: WB Saunders, pp. 875–884.

NOTES

8

Symptom Management and Supportive Care: Rehabilitation and Resources

Doris Ahana

Select the best answer for each of the following questions:

1. Which of the following had the greatest impact in cancer rehabilitation?
   A. JCAHO rehabilitation standards.
   B. Quality of life of cancer survivors.
   C. American Hospital Association patient rights.
   D. Federal Rehabilitation Act of 1973.

2. Rehabilitation emphasizes the _____ of the person with cancer.
   A. functional deficits.
   B. self-care potential.
   C. family limitations.
   D. disease process.

3. Which of the following health care trends affects cancer rehabilitation?
   A. Alternative methods to promote health.
   B. Quality of life issues.
   C. Shift from inpatient to outpatient care.
   D. All of the above.

4. Barriers to cancer rehabilitation include all of the following *except*
   A. public pessimism regarding curability of cancer.
   B. lack of site-specific cancer rehabilitation protocols for clients and families.
   C. lack of available community resources in a managed care environment.
   D. limited reimbursement for rehabilitation services.

5. A comprehensive assessment of the needs of the client with cancer is essential to
   A. establish priorities of rehabilitation activities.
   B. control cost through appropriate resource consumption.
   C. address all dimensions of the individual's needs that affect rehabilitation outcome.
   D. determine which problems require interventions.

6. Which of the following baseline data gathered at the initiation of the rehabilitation program are helpful in evaluating a client's progress?
   A. Social skills.
   B. Personal characteristics.
   C. Learning barriers.
   D. Functional capabilities.

7. In the acute care setting, early identification of the need for consultation with a specific member of the multidisciplinary team should occur at which of the following times?
   A. Definitive treatment plan.
   B. Client and family assessment on admission.
   C. Physician referral to a rehabilitation team member.
   D. Client and family request for assistance.

8. Interdisciplinary planning and care by health professionals is facilitated when there is
   A. a designated coordinator of cancer rehabilitation.
   B. delineation of roles and responsibilities of all team members.
   C. mutual goal setting by client or family and health professionals.
   D. all of the above.

9. The nurse ensures continuity of rehabilitation interventions across settings and caregivers by
   A. completing as much of the family instructions as possible before discharge.
   B. limiting the number of health professionals working with client and family.
   C. helping client and family access and use appropriate rehabilitation services in the community.
   D. communicating informally with health care providers about care.

10. Cancer education helps persons with cancer and their families deal with a diagnosis of cancer. Which one of the following American Cancer Society programs provides cancer education for clients and families?
    A. "I Can Cope" Program.
    B. Encore Exercise program.
    C. Cancer Survivor Celebration of Life.
    D. CanSurmount.

11. The client with cancer of the head and neck who undergoes surgery and subsequent radiation treatment will require
    A. psychosocial resources and support.
    B. nutritional counseling.
    C. speech therapy.
    D. all of the above.

12. Rehabilitation of a client with a new colostomy should include which one of the following nursing actions?
    A. Consult with enterostomal therapist.
    B. Referral to vocational rehabilitation.
    C. Support the client's choice to refuse home care follow-up.
    D. Provide client with essential content to manage the colostomy and give detailed instructions to family.

13. Rehabilitation services for a person with cancer who has completed radiation treatment to the lumbosacral area for relief of pain from metastases include all of the following *except*
    A. implement measures to control pain.
    B. increase mobility using assistive devices.
    C. promote skin care.
    D. prevent urinary incontinence.

14. An organization that provides information and support primarily to clients with breast cancer is
    A. Encore Plus.
    B. Lymphedema Foundation.
    C. The Women's Cancer Network.
    D. Y-Me.

ANSWERS

1. *Answer:* B
   Rationale: Concern for the quality of life of those clients who survive cancer contributes to the growth of cancer rehabilitation. Other responses have no direct influence on the specialty of rehabilitation in cancer.

2. *Answer:* B
   Rationale: Liabilities of client and family are minimized in rehabilitation. Strengths and abilities are emphasized.

3. *Answer:* D
   Rationale: The rise of consumerism in health care has influenced the delivery of cancer rehabilitation. Consumers expect or demand the promotion of wellness and quality of life in different settings. Rehabilitation interventions are initiated and continued on an outpatient basis with early client discharges from the acute setting.

4. *Answer:* B
   Rationale: Site-specific cancer protocols serve as guidelines for the multidisciplinary team. Negative attitudes to cancer prognosis affect the public acceptance of rehabilitation. Gaps in comprehensive rehabilitation services exist because of limited reimbursement and difficulty in securing access to community resources in a managed care environment.

5. *Answer:* C
   Rationale: Rehabilitation addresses all dimensions of the individual (physical, psychological, spiritual, and socioeconomic) to assist the client to achieve optimum function. A, B, and D are not primary reasons for a comprehensive assessment. Those options are considered after initial and ongoing assessment of the comprehensive needs.

6. *Answer:* D
   Rationale: Functional independence is used as a measurement of progress from prehospitalization to discharge. A, B, and C assessment data help to identify individual resources and limitations.

7. *Answer:* B
   Rationale: The nursing admission database triggers cues for further evaluation by other health professionals. Early referrals can then be initiated by the nurse. A, C, and D may not occur on a timely basis.

8. *Answer:* D
   Rationale: All of the options contribute to smooth, efficient, and effective interdisciplinary planning.

9. *Answer:* C
   Rationale: Written instructions versus informal verbal communication promote a continuum of care. Options A and B are unrealistic in view of early client discharges and lack of nurse authority over care providers across the different settings.

10. *Answer:* A
    Rationale: A and D are American Cancer Society–sponsored programs, but only "I Can Cope" provides cancer education classes.

11. *Answer:* D
    Rationale: Responses A, B, and C indicate appropriate health disciplines to handle the potential psychosocial disturbances and functional impairments of speech, chewing, swallowing, and salivary flow with surgery and radiation treatments.

12. *Answer:* A
    Rationale: Consulting the enterostomal therapist on the rehabilitation of clients with new colostomies is essential. Referral to vocational rehabilitation is premature because most clients are able to resume or modify their work. One usually supports or encourages home care follow-up. Education content is the same for the client and family.

13. *Answer:* D
    Rationale: Options A, B, and C support a program of appropriate interventions for palliative rehabilitation. Potential side effects of palliative radiation to the lumbosacral region for the control of pain do not include urinary incontinence.

14. *Answer:* D
    Rationale: Y-Me provides counseling, information, and support groups for breast cancer

clients and families. Other agencies provide information and support to other cancer clients as well.

BIBLIOGRAPHY

Ahana, D. (1998). Symptom management and supportive care: Rehabilitation and resources. In J. Itano & K. Taoka (eds.). *Core Curriculum in Oncology Nursing* (3rd ed.). Philadelphia: WB Saunders, pp. 115–123.

Bedder, S.M., & Aikin, J.L. (1994). Continuity of care: A challenge for ambulatory oncology nursing. *Semin Oncol 10,* 254–263.

Frymark, S. (1992). Rehabilitation resources within the team and community. *Semin Oncol Nurs 8,* 212–218.

Groenwald, S.L., Frogge, J.H., Goodman, M., & Yarbro, C.H. (eds.). (1995). *A Clinical Guide to Cancer Nursing: A Companion to Cancer Nursing.* Boston: Jones & Bartlett, pp. 538–541.

Mellette, S.F., & Blunk, K. (1994). Cancer rehabilitation. *Semin Oncol 21,* 779–782.

Oncology Nursing Society. (1994). *ONS Position Statement on Cancer Rehabilitation.*

Watson, P.G. (1996). Rehabilitation services. In R. McCorkle, M. Grant, M.D. Stromborg, & S.B. Baird (eds.). *Cancer Nursing* (2nd ed.). Philadelphia: WB Saunders, pp. 1300–1311.

NOTES

9

Symptom Management and Supportive Care: Therapies and Procedures

Jan Petree

Select the best answer for each of the following questions:

1. A client asks the nurse if a PICC (peripherally inserted central catheter) line is a good device for intermittent chemotherapy for the next year. The nurse explains to the client all of the following *except*

    A. PICC lines are used for intermediate-term therapy.

    B. the advantages of PICC lines are that there is a decreased risk of infection and a low incidence of thoracic complications, and it can be placed at the bedside.

    C. another device such as a port or tunneled catheter may be more appropriate for intermittent long-term therapy.

    D. PICC lines are cheaper than ports or tunneled catheters, and we are trying to keep costs down.

2. You have been called by a nurse on the medical unit to troubleshoot a client's vascular access device. The patient is 36 years old with acute leukemia and has a double-lumen tunneled catheter. In the large lumen the client is receiving triple antibiotics, blood products, pain medication, and phenytoin (Dilantin) 100 mg q8h. In the small lumen total parenteral nutrition (TPN) (by pump) and lipids 20% (by gravity) were infusing. The large lumen infuses and draws blood without a problem. The small lumen will not in-

fuse or withdraw. The nurse makes which of the following assessments?

    A. A thrombus is most likely present.

    B. A lipid precipitate is most likely present.

    C. Urokinase should be administered.

    D. A Dilantin precipitate is most likely present.

3. The large lumen of the catheter is clogged. You know that the client is receiving blood products, antibiotics, and Dilantin in this lumen. The bag of medication hanging is Dilantin. You are aware that Dilantin precipitates if mixed in any intravenous solution other than normal saline. Normal saline solution is hanging on this line. Nursing actions will be based on the following:

    A. This is most likely a thrombus formation.

    B. Call the physician to remove the vascular access device since drug precipitates cannot be dissolved.

    C. Call the pharmacist to determine the pH of Dilantin. Increase pH with $NaHCO_3$ or decrease pH with hydrochloric acid.

    D. Attempt to flush with dextrose but do not use a syringe smaller than 5 cc because use of 3 cc or 1 cc syringes increases pressure and the catheter could rupture.

4. A physician stops you in the hallway and asks you to insert a catheter in a client who is re-

ceiving nafcillin. You discuss with the physician the following device(s) and recommend the most appropriate device for this patient who is going home for a course of 10 to 14 more days of nafcillin. Which is the best choice?

A. A peripheral line that needs to be changed every 2 to 3 days.
B. A PICC line that can be used for irritating drugs for at least 10 days of therapy.
C. A nontunneled central venous catheter, which can be pulled after therapy.
D. A midline catheter, which is a long arm peripheral line.

5. Which statement is _true_ about potential complications associated with infusion systems?

A. Occlusion, mechanical errors such as a power failure or programming error, and severed tubing are common.
B. Client-controlled infusion systems are difficult for clients to manage.
C. It is uncommon for clients to go home with an infusion system.
D. Clients usually are not anxious about going home with an infusion system.

6. Which of the following statements are _false_ about autologous blood components?

A. It is not recommended that clients donate their own blood before surgery.
B. Red blood cell salvage during surgery is done by automated cell saver devices.
C. Salvaged blood can be returned to the client after surgery.
D. Transfusion services are set up to handle donations of autologous blood several months before surgery.

7. Selecting the type of nutritional therapy (enteral or parenteral) depends on all of the following factors _except_

A. function of gastrointestinal tract.
B. severity of nutritional problem.
C. length of proposed therapy and prognosis.
D. percent of body fat.

8. The preferred method of giving enteral therapy for long-term use is through all of the following _except_

A. a gastrostomy tube.
B. the mouth.
C. a nasogastric tube.
D. a jejunostomy tube.

9. TPN therapy is best administered through which type of vascular access device?

A. Peripheral line.
B. Midline.
C. Central line: PICC, tunneled, or nontunneled.
D. Femoral line.

10. Implanted ports can be placed in peripheral veins, central veins, peritoneal cavity, or the epidural space for pain management. The following statements about implanted ports are all true _except_

A. A vascular port can be placed in the abdomen, and most of the time one obtains a blood return on aspiration.
B. A peritoneal port can be placed in the abdomen, and one may get blood-tinged or clear fluid back on aspiration.
C. An epidural port can be placed in the abdomen, and one usually cannot palpate the tract to the epidural space.
D. An epidural port can be placed in the abdomen, and one will not be able to aspirate fluid unless the port has migrated into the spinal canal.

11. A potential side effect of abruptly stopping TPN is

A. hyperglycemia.
B. hypoglycemia.
C. shaking chills.
D. diarrhea.

12. The _most_ common side effect of administering enteral feedings too rapidly is

A. constipation.
B. vomiting.
C. diarrhea.
D. nausea.

13. One hour after putting urokinase into an occluded central venous catheter, the catheter remains occluded when the nurse attempts to withdraw the urokinase. The nurse should

A. try to force the catheter open with a normal saline solution flush.
B. send the client home with instructions to increase the frequency of heparin flushes.
C. refer the client for insertion of a new catheter.
D. obtain a physician's order for a second dose of urokinase.

14. Twenty-four hours after placement of an implanted port the client presents with regional discomfort, pain, and swelling at the site of the port. The client's vital signs are within normal limits except for a temperature of 37.2° C. Likely problems include all of the following *except*

  A. pocket infection.
  B. port-catheter separation.
  C. venous thrombosis.
  D. trauma to the site.

15. A client with leukemia who recently received high-dose cytarabine presents with a fever and a slightly reddened central venous catheter site. The nurse suspects the fever is *primarily* due to

  A. a possible central venous catheter site infection secondary to chemotherapy-induced neutropenia.
  B. a possible central venous catheter infection secondary to poor catheter exit site care.
  C. a common side effect of cytarabine.
  D. a fast-growing malignancy unresponsive to chemotherapy.

NOTES

ANSWERS

1. *Answer:* D
Rationale: PICC lines are cheaper devices but should not be used for long-term therapy. A port or tunneled catheter would be the most appropriate device.

2. *Answer:* B
Rationale: This is most likely a lipid precipitate. Urokinase dissolves only blood or fibrin clots and would not be helpful in this situation.

3. *Answer:* C
Rationale: Drug precipitates can be dissolved if the staff is aware of the appropriate actions to take. Confirming the pH with the pharmacist and reviewing the policy to dissolve drug precipitates are helpful.

4. *Answer:* B
Rationale: Peripheral lines or midlines are not the vascular access devices of choice because of drug irritation of the peripheral veins. A PICC line would be the line of choice, since central administration of the antibiotic will reduce irritation to peripheral veins.

5. *Answer:* A
Rationale: Occlusion, mechanical errors, and severed tubing are common complications with infusion devices. Clients should have extensive teaching and support from a nurse or pharmacist in the home.

6. *Answer:* A
Rationale: It may be recommended that clients donate their own blood before surgery. There is less risk of contracting an infectious disease from one's own blood.

7. *Answer:* D
Rationale: Obesity has no bearing on the choice of nutrition therapy. Obese clients still need nutritional support.

8. *Answer:* B
Rationale: The mouth is not a good avenue for delivering long-term enteral feedings. Clients usually cannot manage this method successfully and require tube placement.

9. *Answer:* C
Rationale: Parenteral therapy must be administered through a central line because the concentration of dextrose in the solution ranges from 25% to 40%. Peripheral lines and midlines can only handle dextrose solutions of 12% or less because of peripheral vein tolerance. Femoral lines are inconvenient for clients and present a high risk for complications.

10. *Answer:* C
Rationale: Epidural ports can be palpated, and the catheter tract can be followed around to the back.

11. *Answer:* B
Rationale: Insulin production increases with TPN and will halt abruptly if TPN is stopped quickly. With too much insulin, the body reacts by going into hypoglycemia.

12. *Answer:* C
Rationale: Rapid infusion of central feeding overstimulates the gastrointestinal function, and the result is the rapid excretion of the feeding through diarrhea.

13. *Answer:* D
Rationale: If urokinase is not successful after 1 hour, it is recommended that a second dose of urokinase be administered.

14. *Answer:* B
Rationale: Responses A, C, and D could explain the symptoms experienced. A fever would not be indicative of a port-catheter separation.

15. *Answer:* A
Rationale: Catheter exit site infection frequently occurs during the neutropenic phase after chemotherapy.

BIBLIOGRAPHY

Borlase, B.C., Bell, S.J., Blackburn, G.L., et al. (1995). *Enteral Nutrition*. New York: Chapman and Hall.

Cunningham, R.S., & Bonam-Crawford, D. (1993). The role of fibrinolytic agents in the management of thrombotic complications associated with vascular access devices. *Nurs Clin North Am 28*(4), 899–909.

Doane, L.S. (1993). Administering intraperitoneal chemotherapy using a peritoneal port. *Nurs Clin North Am* 28(4), 885–897.

Fischer, J.E. (1991). *Total Parenteral Nutrition* (2nd ed.). Boston: Little, Brown.

Freedman, S.E., & Bosserman, G. (1993). Tunneled catheters: Technologic advances and nursing care issues. *Nurs Clin North Am 28*(4), 851–858.

Gullo, S.M. (1993). Implanted ports: Technologic advances and nursing care issues. *Nurs Clin North Am 28*(4), 859–871.

Merrick, H.W. (1995). Vascular access, infusion, and perfusion. In R.T. Skeel (ed.). *Handbook of Cancer Chemotherapy* (4th ed.). Boston: Little, Brown, pp. 680–688.

Ryder, M.A. (1993). Peripherally inserted central venous catheters. *Nurs Clin North Am 28*(4), 937–971.

Wile, A. (1996). Indications and devices for chronic venous access. In S.E. Wilson (ed.). *Vascular Access: Principles and Practice* (3rd ed.). St. Louis: Mosby, pp. 54–58.

NOTES

10

Symptom Management and Supportive Care: Pharmacologic Interventions

Carolyn S. J. Ma and Karen N. Taoka

Select the best answer for each of the following questions:

1. Mrs. J. has breast cancer and is being treated with chemotherapy. The white blood cell count 10 days after her last treatment is 800. Her physician prescribes prophylactic antibiotics to be given at home. Which is an appropriate statement for you to teach Mrs. J.?
   A. Discontinue daily temperature monitoring during antibiotic therapy.
   B. Take all daily antibiotic doses between 8 AM and 5 PM.
   C Notify the physician of any rash, fever, or nausea.
   D. Chills are an expected side effect of antibiotic therapy.

2. Amphotericin B and fluconazole are two common agents used for the treatment of
   A. *Staphylococcus.*
   B. *Candida albicans.*
   C. *Streptococcus.*
   D. *Escherichia coli.*

3. Aminoglycosides are used in conjunction with other antimicrobials to treat infections in clients with cancer. The major toxicity of aminoglycosides is
   A. hepatotoxicity.
   B. cardiac toxicity.
   C. nephrotoxicity.
   D. neurotoxicity.

4. Acyclovir is commonly used to treat
   A. *Pseudomonas* pneumonia.
   B. herpes simplex infection.
   C. pulmonary aspergillosis.
   D. cytomegalovirus retinitis.

5. Mrs. C. is receiving cefazolin sodium for an *E. coli* infection. The nurse teaching Mrs. C. and her family regarding signs and symptoms of hypersensitivity reactions would instruct them to observe for all of the following *except*
   A. shortness of breath.
   B. appearance of hives.
   C. increased urine output.
   D. a fast heart rate.

6. Nonsteroidal antiinflammatory agents suppress the inflammatory response by
   A. inhibiting cyclooxygenase and the production of prostaglandins.
   B. blocking opiate neurotransmitters.
   C. causing tumor cell lysis.
   D. increasing macrophage migration to the site of injury.

7. Mr. T. has coronary artery disease and takes one aspirin daily. He has recently had a diagnosis of metastatic lung cancer, and the physician has prescribed naproxen sodium and dexamethasone for bone pain. Mr. T. is at higher risk for the following side effects *except*
   A. gastrointestinal ulceration.
   B. bleeding.

C. fluid retention and renal insufficiency.

D. constipation.

8. A 16-year-old female has osteosarcoma with bone pain. She will be receiving a corticosteroid indefinitely. Client teaching should include discussion of which of the following side effects?

A. Acne, weight gain, and moon face.

B. Altered mental alertness.

C. Amenorrhea.

D. Loss of appetite.

9. All of the following chemotherapeutic agents have a high emetogenic potential *except*

A. cisplatin.

B. paclitaxel.

C. mechlorethamine.

D. dacarbazine.

10. Nursing actions when administering serotonin antagonists include

A. administering diphenhydramine to prevent extrapyramidal symptoms (EPS).

B. monitoring vital signs for hypertension.

C. administering acetaminophen for headache.

D. teaching clients to take only as needed (prn) for nausea, vomiting.

11. The advantage of serotonin antagonists over substituted benzamides and phenothiazines is

A. cost.

B. lack of EPS.

C. sedation.

D. anticholinergic effects.

12. The following drugs are often given to augment antiemetics *except*

A. diphenhydramine.

B. diazepam.

C. lorazepam.

D. cimetidine.

13. The rationale for the use of lorazepam and diazepam to augment antiemetics includes

A. the additional blockade of serotonin.

B. the additional blockade of dopamine.

C. causing anterograde amnesia.

D. central action inhibits the vomiting center.

14. Mr. D. will be receiving high-dose cisplatin at 100 mg/m^2 intravenously for lung cancer.

Principles of nursing management for antiemetic therapy would include all of the following *except*

A. administering serotonin antagonists before the cisplatin.

B. administering antiemetics on a scheduled basis.

C. administering antiemetic only when Mr.

D. vomits.

D. administering adjuvant antiemetics as necessary to control breakthrough nausea and vomiting.

15. Which of the following analgesics is more likely to cause respiratory depression?

A. Hydromorphone hydrochloride.

B. Buprenorphine hydrochloride.

C. Pentazocine.

D. Acetaminophen.

16. Side effects of opioid analgesics include all of the following *except*

A. respiratory depression.

B. visual and auditory hallucinations.

C. diarrhea.

D. urinary retention.

17. Nursing interventions to assist the client with cancer to deal with the gastrointestinal side effects of opioid analgesics include all of the following *except*

A. restricting fluids.

B. increasing dietary fiber intake.

C. monitoring bowel sounds.

D. administering stool softeners/stimulants.

18. When administering morphine sustained-release tablets to a client through a nasogastric feeding tube, the nurse should

A. crush the tablets and administer concurrently with the tube feeding.

B. clamp the tube for 30 minutes, crush the tablets, and then administer.

C. find an alternative route of administration (e.g., intrarectally or vaginally).

D. crush the tablets and add to tube feeding solution.

19. Mr. C. is taking aspirin for rheumatoid arthritis and is also receiving 5-FU, doxorubicin, and methotrexate for colon cancer. What risk

may be significantly increased as a result of drug interaction?

    A. Increased risk for cardiac toxicity.
    B. Increased risk of methotrexate toxicity.
    C. Increased risk for diarrhea.
    D. Increased risk for aspirin toxicity.

20. Mrs. C. is being discharged while taking hydrocodone and acetaminophen. Which of the following is *not* a discharge instruction for this medication?

    A. Take the amount prescribed.
    B. Increase fluid and fiber intake to prevent constipation.
    C. Use of alcohol will not cause excessive drowsiness.
    D. Avoid driving or other hazardous activities that require mental alertness.

21. A common drug used as an antianxiety agent is

    A. flurazepam.
    B. secobarbital.
    C. phenytoin.
    D. alprazolam.

22. A major disadvantage of using barbiturates as a sedative/hypnotic agent is

    A. rebound anxiety.
    B. loss of concentration and depression of affect.
    C. tolerance builds quickly.
    D. high incidence of Stevens-Johnson syndrome.

23. Mrs. H. is 82 years old with lung cancer and bone metastases for which she is given dexamethasone and morphine. She received flurazepam two nights in a row for insomnia because of increased pain at night. On the third day she is difficult to arouse, disoriented, and confused. All of the following are possible reasons for the central nervous system (CNS) symptoms *except* that

    A. flurazepam is one of the longest-acting benzodiazepine sedative/hypnotic agents.
    B. flurazepam may potentiate the CNS depressant side effects of morphine.
    C. flurazepam and dexamethasone work synergistically to increase CNS depressant side effects.
    D. Mrs. H. is elderly.

24. A better alternative for Mrs. H. is

    A. triazolam.
    B. phenobarbital.
    C. chlordiazepoxide HCl.
    D. diazepam.

25. A frequent side effect of haloperidol is

    A. orthostatic hypotension.
    B. extrapyramidal symptoms.
    C. urinary retention.
    D. sedation.

26. Indications for use of antidepressants in cancer patients include all of the following *except*

    A. depression.
    B. adjuvant pain management.
    C. to counteract sedation.
    D. pain from postherpetic neuralgia.

27. In a patient with brain metastases, phenytoin (Dilantin) may be a necessary prophylactic medication if the patient is receiving which of the following drugs?

    A. Granisetron and dexamethasone.
    B. Prochlorperazine and meperidine.
    C. Acetaminophen and codeine.
    D. Naproxen sodium and dexamethasone.

28. The following is *true* about hematopoietic growth factors (HGFs). They

    A. exert biological effects such as enhancing differentiation or maturation of immunologic cell lines.
    B. promote tumor activity by stimulating bone marrow stem cells.
    C. are used for primary treatment of breast cancer.
    D. do not affect duration of neutropenia.

29. A common side effect of G-CSF is

    A. sedation.
    B. bone pain.
    C. diarrhea.
    D. constipation.

30. Common side effects of high dose GM-CSF include the following *except*

    A. pericardial effusions.
    B. capillary leak syndrome.
    C. hepatic insufficiency.
    D. third spacing of fluids.

31. Nursing actions when administering HGFs include all of the following *except*
    A. knowing intravenous HGFs may require albumin in the carrier solution.
    B. administering acetaminophen for bone pain.
    C. shaking the vial vigorously during reconstitution.
    D. rotating the sites of injection for subcutaneous injections.

32. G-CSF acts by
    A. decreasing phagocytic activity.
    B. stimulating precursors committed to neutrophil lineage.
    C. interacting with specific receptors on erythroid burst-forming units.
    D. regulating megakaryocytopoiesis.

33. Mr. L. immigrated to the United States from Hong Kong 3 years ago and speaks limited English. He is 57 years old, has lung cancer, and is seen in a clinic in Chinatown for his chemotherapy. After seeking a traditional Chinese herbalist to treat his anxiety, Mr. L. turned to his Western physician who prescribed diazepam for him. In Chinese clients receiving diazepam, which of the following may apply?
    A. Mr. L. probably needs a lower dose of diazepam.
    B. All Chinese herbs interact with diazepam.
    C. Mr. L. should increase the dose of diazepam as needed.
    D. Mr. L. should take the diazepam with tea.

34. Nursing considerations when caring for multicultural clientele include all of the following *except*
    A. an awareness that herbal preparations may have adverse interactions with prescribed medications.
    B. clients from different cultural and ethnic backgrounds routinely consult with traditional healers.
    C. biological variations among racial groups may affect drug metabolism rates, clinical drug responses, and side effects to drugs.
    D. health care practices and beliefs influence self-medicating behaviors of clients.

NOTES

ANSWERS

1. *Answer:* C
Rationale: Rash, fever, and nausea may indicate a reaction to the antibiotic or may indicate another infectious process. The physician would need to be aware of these symptoms to treat the client properly.

2. *Answer:* B
Rationale: These are antifungal agents and *Candida* is a fungal organism.

3. *Answer:* C
Rationale: The major toxicity of aminoglycosides is nephrotoxicity. Careful monitoring of antibiotic levels (peak and trough), serum creatinine levels, and urine output is indicated to maximize treatment while minimizing toxicity.

4. *Answer:* B
Rationale: Acyclovir is an antiviral agent indicated in the treatment of herpes simplex virus and varicella zoster virus. *Pseudomonas* pneumonia is a bacterial infection. Pulmonary aspergillosis is a fungal infection. Acyclovir is not effective against cytomegalovirus retinitis.

5. *Answer:* C
Rationale: Hypersensitivity reactions to cephalosporins may decrease urinary output.

6. *Answer:* A
Rationale: The mechanism of action of nonsteroidal antiinflammatory agents involves the inhibition of cyclooxygenase and thus the production of prostaglandins. This break in the cascade in turn suppresses the inflammatory response of white blood cell and macrophage migration to the site of injury and results in or contributes to symptom relief. Antiinflammatory agents do not work centrally by blocking opiate neurotransmitters and do not cause tumor cell lysis.

7. *Answer:* D
Rationale: The combined interaction and potential side effects of aspirin, naproxen sodium, and dexamethasone put Mr. T. at higher risk of gastrointestinal ulceration, bleeding, and fluid retention and urinary insufficiency. Constipation is not a common side effect.

8. *Answer:* A
Rationale: Acne, weight gain, moon face, and an increase in appetite are common side effects of corticosteroids. For a teenage girl especially, these side effects will more than likely affect her body image. Amenorrhea and central nervous system sedation are not common side effects of corticosteroids.

9. *Answer:* B
Rationale: Paclitaxel has a low emetogenic potential. Cisplatin, mechlorethamine, and dacarbazine all have a high emetogenic potential.

10. *Answer:* C
Rationale: Headache is a common side effect of serotonin antagonists. EPS and hypertension are not usual side effects of serotonin antagonists. A prn administration schedule is contraindicated for serotonin antagonists.

11. *Answer:* B
Rationale: Serotonin antagonists, although more expensive than substituted benzamides and phenothiazines, do not have EPS as a notable adverse side effect. However, sedation and anticholinergic effects may occur.

12. *Answer:* D
Rationale: Diphenhydramine, diazepam, and lorazepam are all often used to augment antiemetics. Cimetidine is an H_2 blocker that is not indicated for augmentation of antiemetics.

13. *Answer:* C
Rationale: By causing anterograde amnesia, lorazepam and diazepam lessen the negative experience of nausea and vomiting by effectively blocking a "memory" of this unpleasant experience. This, in turn, helps to decrease the incidence of anticipatory nausea and vomiting. The other choices are not actions of lorazepam and diazepam.

14. *Answer:* C
Rationale: Principles of nursing management include the administration of antiemetics prophylactically to cover the onset, peak, and duration of action of each antineoplastic agent.

Waiting to administer antiemetics only when a client vomits is not recommended.

15. *Answer:* A

Rationale: Buprenorphine hydrochloride and pentazocine are agonist-antagonist compounds and less likely to cause respiratory depression than hydromorphone hydrochloride.

16. *Answer:* C

Rationale: Diarrhea is not a side effect of opioid analgesics; constipation is usually associated with opioid analgesics.

17. *Answer:* A

Rationale: Constipation is a common gastrointestinal side effect of opioid analgesics; restricting fluids would aggravate this side effect. All of the other answers are interventions to prevent constipation.

18. *Answer:* C

Rationale: Finding an alternative route is the best solution because any of the other options involving tube feeding can compromise pain relief by increasing transit time and decreasing gastrointestinal absorption of the tablets. Sustained-release tablets cannot be crushed.

19. *Answer:* B

Rationale: Aspirin competes with methotrexate for protein binding sites, thus liberating methotrexate into the circulation.

20. *Answer:* C

Rationale: Alcohol enhances the CNS depressant side effects of hydrocodone.

21. *Answer:* D

Rationale: Flurazepam and secobarbital are sedative-hypnotic agents. Phenytoin is an anticonvulsant.

22. *Answer:* C

Rationale: Stevens-Johnson syndrome does occur, but it is rare. Rebound anxiety and loss of concentration and depression of affect are not usual side effects of barbiturates.

23. *Answer:* C

Rationale: Flurazepam and dexamethasone do not work synergistically to increase CNS side effects. One of the side effects of dexamethasone is CNS stimulation. The other answers are correct since flurazepam is one of the longest acting benzodiazepines and its side effects may persist for days after administration. It can also potentiate the CNS depressant side effects of morphine. Elderly clients are more sensitive to CNS depressant side effects of drugs.

24. *Answer:* A

Rationale: Triazolam is a short-acting sedative-hypnotic agent with minimal daytime hangover effect. Chlordiazepoxide HCl and diazepam are indicated more for anxiety, seizure control, and alcohol withdrawal. Phenobarbital is a long-acting sedative.

25. *Answer:* B

Rationale: EPS is a side effect frequently associated with haloperidol. Orthostatic hypotension, urinary retention, and sedation occur infrequently.

26. *Answer:* C

Rationale: Depression, adjuvant pain management, and postherpetic neuralgia are all indications for antidepressant use in clients with cancer. Some antidepressants may cause sedation.

27. *Answer:* B

Rationale: Neither granisetron and dexamethasone nor naproxen sodium and dexamethasone lower the seizure threshold. Although codeine may lower the seizure threshold, B is the best answer since prochlorperazine lowers the seizure threshold and normeperidine (the metabolite of meperidine) may also lower the seizure threshold.

28. *Answer:* A

Rationale: HGFs do not promote tumor activity by stimulating bone marrow stem cells. They are not used as a primary treatment for breast cancer, and they can shorten the duration of neutropenia.

29. *Answer:* B

Rationale: Sedation, diarrhea, and constipation are not common side effects of G-CSF. Bone pain is a common side effect.

30. *Answer:* C

Rationale: Hepatic insufficiency is not a common side effect of high-dose GM-CSF therapy. All of the other side effects are common with high-dose GM-CSF treatment.

31. *Answer:* C
   Rationale: Vigorous shaking of the vial is contraindicated, since this can denature the protein.

32. *Answer:* B
   Rationale: G-CSF increases phagocytic activity. It does not interact with the erythroid or platelet cell lines.

33. *Answer:* A
   Rationale: Because of biological variations, the Chinese have been found to require a lower dose of benzodiazepines and are more sensitive to the sedative effects of this drug class.

34. *Answer:* B
   Rationale: Although traditional healers are frequently consulted, it cannot be assumed that clients will always consult these healers.

BIBLIOGRAPHY

Bociek, R.G., & Armitage, J.O. (1996). Hematopoietic growth factors. *CA Cancer J Clin 46*(3), 165–184.

Cleri, L.B. (1995). Serotonin antagonists: State of the art management of chemotherapy-induced emesis. *Oncology Nursing: Patient Treatment and Support 2*(1), 1–20.

DiGregorio, G.J., Barbieri, E.J., Sterling, G.H., Camp, J.F., & Prout, M.F. (1994). *Handbook of Pain Management* (4th ed.). West Chester, PA: Medical Surveillance.

Dorr, R.T., & Van Horn, D. (1994). *Cancer Chemotherapy Handbook* (2nd ed.). Norwalk, CT: Appleton & Lange.

Malseed, R.T., Goldstein, F.J., & Balkon, N. (1995). *Pharmacology: Drug Therapy and Nursing Considerations* (4th ed.). Philadelphia: JB Lippincott.

Pitler, L.R. (1996). Hematopoietic growth factors in clinical practice. *Semin Oncol Nurs 12*(2), 115–129.

Rhodes, V.A., Johnson, M.H., & McDaniel, R.W. (1995). Nausea, vomiting, and retching: The management of the symptom experience. *Semin Oncol Nurs 11*(4), 256–265.

Skidmore-Roth, L. (1996). *Mosby's Nursing Drug Reference.* St. Louis: Mosby–Year Book.

NOTES

PART II

Protective Mechanisms

11

Alterations in Mobility, Skin Integrity, and Neurologic Status

Jennifer Douglas Pearce

Select the best answer for each of the following questions:

1. Mr. R., a 50-year-old construction worker, is admitted to rule out prostate cancer. On interview, he states that he has been in bed for the past 3 weeks because of lower back pain. Mr. R. has an alteration in mobility related to
   A. osseous involvement and nerve compression.
   B. side effects from steroid therapy.
   C. side effects from radiation therapy.
   D. altered or decreased nutritional intake.

2. A client presents with right-sided hemiparesis.. There is a decrease in muscle tone. Which of the following nursing diagnoses would be a priority to include in the plan of care?
   A. Alteration in mobility related to paralysis.
   B. Alteration in bowel elimination related to paralysis.
   C. Self-care deficit related to limitations of movement.
   D. Alterations in skin integrity related to decrease in tissue perfusion.

3. A client with multiple myeloma would demonstrate a knowledge deficit of the disease process if which of the following occurs?
   A. The client decreases ambulation with bone pain.
   B. The client increases fluid intake.

C. The client avoids heavy lifting.
D. The client monitors serum calcium.

4. Which of the following is a correctly stated nursing diagnosis for a client with vision and hearing deficits related to chemotherapy?
   A. Pain related to side effects of therapy.
   B. Anxiety and fear related to potential or actual loss of senses.
   C. High risk for altered tissue perfusion related to decrease in cerebral blood flow.
   D. High risk for alteration in skin integrity related to decrease in cerebral blood flow.

5. Mrs. H. has breast cancer that has metastasized to the spinal cord. Passive range of motion is ordered for her impaired physical mobility. The nurse understands that
   A. passive range of motion exercises increase muscle strength.
   B. range of motion requires full participation by the client.
   C. exercise should be completed to the point of discomfort.
   D. range of motion exercise is beneficial to carry out activities of daily living.

6. A client with a history of poor nutrition after chemotherapy is admitted to the hospital. Which of the following nursing measures would be

most appropriate to maintain the integrity of the client's skin?

- A. Encourage client to change position every 2 hours.
- B. Place sheepskin pads on client's heels and elbows.
- C. Encourage client to get up in a chair at least 3 hours a day.
- D. Have client lie in a prone position.

7. The nursing assessment of a client with an order for passive range of motion exercise should include all of the following *except*

- A. general condition assessment.
- B. establishing range of motion function before present condition.
- C. taking baseline vital signs.
- D. encouraging the client to communicate presence of pain during exercise.

Situation: Mrs. G., age 34, is admitted to rule out lung cancer. She has a nursing diagnosis of ineffective individual coping and is experiencing a severe anxiety reaction.

8. She greets the nurse by saying, "People come to the hospital to get better. But you people are so inefficient and noisy, I can't get any rest around here!" Which is your best response?

- A. "What is it about the staff that you don't like?"
- B. "You feel frightened and anxious about being in the hospital."
- C. "Let me explain our routine. I am sure you will understand the staff a little better."
- D. "I agree. At times we are a bit disorganized. Maybe you could help."

9. You are preparing for a team conference for Mrs. G. The goal is for Mrs. G. to demonstrate positive self-efficacy. You formulate the following expected outcomes; the client will

- A. gain insight into the cause of her anxiety.
- B. recognize that behavior is related to anxiety.
- C. increase her tolerance for coping with anxiety.
- D. verbalize new ways of coping with anxiety.

10. As Mrs. G.'s nurse, you find that you experience some irritation while working with her. The attitude to maintain while working with her is

- A. a matter-of-fact approach.
- B. willingness to help her in everything.
- C. calm and supportive.
- D. light and amusing.

11. A client who had a mastectomy is in her third week of radiation therapy. You note that her skin appears wet and weeping. Your intervention is to

- A. withhold radiation treatment and explain that the client must not bathe until the weeping has stopped.
- B. send her for the radiation treatment as ordered and make a note on her treatment record.
- C. consult the physician before continuing radiation treatment.
- D. send her for the radiation treatment and instruct the client to use lotion on the area.

Situation: The client, Ms R., age 90 years, has a nursing diagnosis of alteration in mental status after chemotherapy.

12. Which of the following statements provide the most appropriate reality orientation for Ms R. when she first awakens in the morning?

- A. "Do you remember who I am or what day it is today?"
- B. "Hello, Ms R. Did you sleep well? Which dress would you like to wear today, the green or the yellow?"
- C. "Here I am again, Ms R. Today is Tuesday so there will be pancakes for breakfast this morning."
- D. Good morning, Ms R. This is your second day in St. Ruth's Hospital and I am your nurse for today. My name is Ms P."

13. Which of the following interventions should be included in the client's plan of care?

- A. Have two assistive personnel follow her when she is up and about.
- B. Remove all objects from her path that client can trip over.
- C. Put her belongings in a safe place, so that she will not lose them.
- D. Give her medications in liquid form to ensure that they are swallowed.

14. Nursing orders would include diversional activity and would be most appropriately di-

rected toward giving Ms R. a chance to do which of the following?
- A. Succeed at a task.
- B. Compete with others.
- C. Socialize with others.
- D. Concentrate on a task.

15. Ms R. has sleep balance disturbance. At nighttime she walks the halls and complains of difficulty getting to sleep. An appropriate nursing intervention to add to the plan of care is
- A. a daily afternoon nap to prevent over-tiredness at night.
- B. administration of a hypnotic drug at bedtime.
- C. active exercise daily so she will be comfortably tired at night.
- D. a cup of hot tea with lemon before bed to promote a feeling of well-being.

16. Which of the following interventions related to activities of daily living would *not* be appropriate for Ms R.?
- A. Make demands on her ability.
- B. Monitor her fluid intake and output.
- C. Arouse strong positive feelings in her.
- D. Change her physical surroundings occasionally.

17. Ms R.'s daughter states that her mother has worn the same wornout, dirty undergarment for weeks at home. Which of the following interventions would be most appropriate for the nursing staff to follow to decrease the risk of regression in Ms R.'s personal hygiene habits?
- A. Accept her need to go without bathing if she so desires.
- B. Have the patient assume responsibility for all physical care.
- C. Make her do as much self-care as she is capable of doing.
- D. Do most of her physical care while letting her think she did it herself.

Situation: Mr. J., a 76-year-old client who is hard of hearing, is receiving radiation therapy for prostate cancer with bone metastases.

18. Mr. J.'s x-ray film shows no shoulder involvement; however, he complains of shoulder stiffness. Which of the following activities of daily living should the client be encouraged to

perform to decrease the risk of loss of shoulder motion?
- A. Shaving himself.
- B. Feeding himself.
- C. Combing his hair.
- D. Cleaning his dentures.

19. Mr. J. is on bed rest. The nurse discovers that Mr. J. has a 26-year history of smoking. A preventive measure to decrease the client's risk of developing alterations in respiratory function is to
- A. have him deep breathe and cough every 1 to 2 hours.
- B. have him wear elastic stockings.
- C. place him in a semisitting position frequently.
- D. encourage him to drink at least 1,500 mL of fluids daily.

20. Mrs. M. had a right mastectomy. She has returned from the recovery room to her room on the medical-surgical oncology unit. Which is the best position for Mrs. M.'s right arm as you position her in bed?
- A. Place her arm across her chest wall.
- B. Place her arm at her side at the same level as her body.
- C. Place her arm in the position that affords her the greatest comfort.
- D. Place her arm on pillows with her hand higher than her elbow and her elbow higher than her shoulder.

21. The nurse teaches Ms P. that a normal tissue response to radiation most often appears as
- A. atrophy of the skin.
- B. scattered pustule formation.
- C. redness of the surface tissue.
- D. sloughing of two layers of the skin.

Situation: Mr. V. has been in a semiconscious state and on bed rest for the past 6 months since a craniotomy for a brain tumor. Two of his high-risk nursing diagnoses are high risk for alteration in skin integrity and high risk for impaired physical mobility.

22. To prevent external rotation of Mr. V.'s hips while he is lying on his back, it would be appropriate for the nurse to place
- A. a firm pillow under the length of his legs.
- B. sandbags alongside his legs from knees to ankles.

C. trochanter rolls alongside his legs from ilium to midthigh.

D. a footboard that supports his feet in the normal anatomic position.

23. At which of the bony prominences does Mr. V. have the least potential for developing a decubitus ulcer?

A. The heels.

B. The knees.

C. The coccyx.

D. The back of the head.

Situation: Mr. K. has alterations in physical mobility related to right-sided weakness secondary to a central nervous system brain tumor.

24. Mr. K. requires oral hygiene at regular intervals. Which of the following techniques used by the nurse is *inappropriate?* The nurse

A. places the client on his back with a small pillow under his head.

B. has portable suction equipment in readiness at the bedside.

C. opens the client's mouth with a padded tongue blade.

D. cleans the client's mouth and teeth with a toothbrush.

25. Mr. K. is at risk for developing decubitus ulcers. What color is the skin when pressure is *first* applied?

A. Bluish.

B. Reddish.

C. Whitish.

D. Yellowish.

26. Mr. K. has impaired communication related to damage to the left side of the brain secondary to CNS neoplasm. The *least helpful* intervention to facilitate communication between the client and the nurse is for the nurse to

A. converse in a slow manner.

B. use gestures to accompany the spoken word.

C. give directions one at a time.

D. speak in a louder than usual tone of voice.

27. Mr. K. is entering the rehabilitation phase and is aware of and discouraged by his physical impairments. The nurse helps him overcome this negative self-concept by demonstrating an attitude of

A. helpfulness with sympathy.

B. concern with charitableness.

C. direction while displaying firmness.

D. positive reinforcement with patience.

Situation: The client at high risk for impaired physical immobility is reluctant to move in bed or to get out of bed.

28. The client's inactivity will affect all of the physiologic functions *except*

A. storage of vitamin B_{12} in the liver.

B. production and excretion of urine.

C. movement of gases and fluid in the lungs.

D. movement of content in the gastrointestinal tract.

29. The client's musculoskeletal system is to be examined. Which of the following tests should the nurse anticipate will be used to provide the information?

A. Synovial fluid analysis.

B. Radioactive isotope skeletal surveys.

C. Blood sedimentation rate and red blood cell count.

D. Serum and urine calcium and phosphorus levels.

30. Which lifestyle changes should the client make to decrease the risk of constipation?

A. Decreased activity level.

B. High-fiber diet.

C. High laxative usage.

D. Low fluid intake.

Situation: Mrs. G. has had a modified radical mastectomy.

31. To decrease the postoperative lymphedema of the affected arm, which of the following should Mrs. G. do?

A. Elevate her arm on pillows above heart level.

B. Keep arm fixed over surgical site.

C. Apply a warm pad over the affected arm.

D. Use only the unaffected arm for all activities.

32. Which of the following exercises is the most appropriate for Mrs. G. to do on the first postoperative day?
    A. Abduction of the affected arm and flexion of the elbow.
    B. "Wall walking" exercises every 4 hours.
    C. Using a rope pulley for extension of the shoulders.
    D. Washing her face using the affected arm.

33. Mrs. G. asks if she should still do monthly breast self-examinations. Which of the following would be the best response by the nurse?
    A. "Yes, to note changes in the affected arm."
    B. "No, there is no further risk of breast cancer."
    C. "No, the doctor will do it every 3 months."
    D. "Yes, there is an increased risk of cancer in the other breast."

34. Mr. H.'s mobility is limited because he experiences dyspnea with minimal exertion. Which of the following pulmonary function findings should the nurse expect to observe?
    A. Increased expiratory times.
    B. Normal ventilation/perfusion ratio.
    C. Normal forced expiratory volume.
    D. Decreased residual volume.

Situation: Mrs. M. is admitted for a below-the-knee amputation as a result of an osteogenic sarcoma.

35. Which of the following interventions would best meet Mrs. M.'s mobility needs after a below-the-knee amputation?
    A. Assist Mrs. M. to stay out of bed as long as possible.
    B. Elevate the residual right limb on a pillow continuously.
    C. Teach her to lift 5-pound weights with her arms.
    D. Provide passive range of motion exercises to the unaffected leg.

36. Mrs. M. is participating in stump wrapping because she has a goal of complete independence in all activities of daily living. The nurse should inform her that the goal of the activity is to
    A. provide range of motion for upper extremities as well as the residual limb.
    B. keep the residual limb clean and dry.
    C. improve muscle tone in the residual limb.
    D. shape the stump for the prosthesis.

37. In instructing Mr. F. about self-care while he is receiving radiation therapy to the oral cavity, which of the following statements would indicate a need for further teaching?
    A. "Since my friend told me about honey in limebud tea, my mouth feels less dry and sticky."
    B. "I'm going to throw out my Cepacol and start using baking soda and water."
    C. "So much for my scotch and soda before dinner."
    D. "I guess I better get these dentures checked. They've been bothering me since I lost all that weight."

38. A 52-year-old woman with breast cancer reports itching. Which of the following could increase the severity of her pruritus?
    A. Anticholinergics.
    B. Hypercalcemia.
    C. Antihistamines.
    D. Hydration.

39. Which of the following interventions would be included in self-care instructions for a client with pruritus?
    A. Take frequent, warm baths to promote vasodilation.
    B. Use petroleum-based lubricants on your skin.
    C. Avoid cutaneous stimulation at the site of itching.
    D. Use water-based lubricants on your skin.

40. In teaching Mrs. O. about her continuous fluorouracil infusion, you have included instructions about the importance of an oral care protocol. These instructions include
    A. perform an assessment of the oral cavity on a weekly basis.
    B. remove white patches gently if present on your tongue or mouth and apply a lanolin-based gel.
    C. begin a low-residue, semisoft diet to prevent stomatitis.
    D. call your doctor immediately if white patches appear on your tongue or mouth.

41. Which of the following interventions would be recommended for a client with the nursing diagnosis high risk for alteration in oral mucous membranes related to side effects of 5-fluorouracil?
    A. Schedule oral care for q2h with a soft toothbrush and nonfluoridated abrasive dentifrice to remove debris.
    B. Rinse mouth q2h while awake and q4h during the night with baking soda and peroxide rinse.
    C. Schedule oral care with a soft toothbrush, fluoridated toothpaste with baking soda, and isotonic sodium chloride solution for q2–4h while awake.
    D. Continue with current oral care—twice-a-day brushing and rinsing with commercial rinses until stomatitis actually develops.

42. Nursing care for the client with bone metastasis and hypercalcemia should include which of the following measures?
    A. Providing a high-protein, low-sodium diet.
    B. Limiting mobility, providing a high-caloric diet.
    C. Increasing hydration, increasing mobility.
    D. Limiting fluid intake, monitoring output.

43. Which of the following nursing diagnoses is *not* appropriate for a woman with breast cancer and bone metastasis?
    A. High risk for alteration in mental status.
    B. High risk for alteration in skin integrity.
    C. High risk for alteration in hygiene.
    D. High risk for injury.

44. Mrs. S. has breast cancer with metastasis to the bone. She is at risk for hypercalcemia. Which of the following assessments would indicate an initial clinical symptom of hypercalcemia?
    A. Respiratory rate.
    B. Muscle tone.
    C. Mental status.
    D. Urinary output.

45. Mrs. C. is being treated with high-volume saline infusions for hypercalcemia (Ca = 14.5 mg/dL). Which of the following interventions would be critical in providing safe care for Mrs. C.?
    A. Encourage Mrs. C. to ask for help when ambulating to the bathroom.
    B. Measure urine output after every void.

C. Assist Mrs. C. to a bedside commode every 2 hours.
D. Clean and dry the perineum after each void.

46. Mr. J., a client with colon cancer, returns for his clinic appointment. His sclera are jaundiced and he has an enlarged abdomen. His wife states that he has been acting strangely lately. He is sleeping more and when awake has periods of confusion. The most likely cause of his symptoms is
    A. sepsis.
    B. narcotic toxicity.
    C. hepatic failure.
    D. hypoxia.

47. In assessing Mr. J., the nurse is aware that signs and symptoms of progressive delirium do not include
    A. confusion.
    B. withdrawal.
    C. agitation.
    D. hallucinations.

48. Mrs. B. has spinal cord compression due to breast cancer. A nursing priority to maintain the nutritional status of Mrs. B. in the presence of impaired physical mobility should include all of the following *except*
    A. oral hygiene before meals.
    B. social isolation during meal time.
    C. position of comfort for eating.
    D. appropriate temperature of food.

49. The rationale for establishing a routine for ADL with Mrs. B., who has impaired physical mobility, is to
    A. reinforce behaviors that are positive.
    B. encourage the client's involvement with ADL.
    C. allow verbalization of feelings and anxieties.
    D. increase understanding of treatment regimen.

50. A client experiencing cognitive dysfunction is taught all of the following *except* to
    A. have periods of uninterrupted sleep.
    B. avoid activities that precipitate fatigue.
    C. self-administer medications.
    D. report feelings of anxiety to a family member.

51. The appropriate time for the nurse to provide client and family education regarding the neurotoxic effects of chemotherapeutic agents is
   A. when the client requests it.
   B. before the treatment.
   C. as the symptoms appear.
   D. after the physician has requested client education.

52. The nurse is assessing a client's neurosensory cerebellar function. The client has a history of neuropathy after chemotherapy. Which of the following assessment techniques is correct?
   A. Test the deep-tendon reflexes to observe for weakness.
   B. Check for pupillary constriction.
   C. Observe erect posture, arm swing, and brisk gait.
   D. Have client smile and stick tongue out.

53. A priority of care when a client is receiving chemotherapy is for the nurse to assess for deep tendon reflexes. The nurse can assess
   A. the extent to which the client is adhering to the prescribed exercise program.
   B. the improvement in the deep tendon reflex response.

C. the presence of neuropathies for modification of the chemotherapy regimen.
   D. strong deep tendon reflexes, which indicate the chemotherapy is combating target cells effectively.

54. Nonpharmacologic interventions for a client experiencing peripheral neuropathy due to chemotherapy include all of the following *except*
   A. progressive muscle relaxation.
   B. guided imagery and massage.
   C. location application of ice packs.
   D. administration of phenytoin chloride.

55. Mr. L. recently has been diagnosed with AIDS-related dementia and secondary lymphoma. In preparing Mr. L. for discharge, all of the following would be appropriate to include in teaching *except* to
   A. keep clocks, calendars, and night lights handy.
   B. restrict social contact to members of the family only.
   C. make an activity list.
   D. keep routines simple and consistent.

ANSWERS

1. **Answer:** A
   Rationale: Client may have widespread disease with bone and neuritic pain due to osseous involvement or nerve compression. Option B is incorrect because there is no indication that a treatment regimen has been implemented at this time. Option C (radiation treatments) may cause fatigue, which can impair physical mobility. Option D is incorrect.

2. **Answer:** D
   Rationale: A leading cause of skin breakdown is a decrease in tissue perfusion due to lack of oxygenation. Options A, B, and C are important but not a priority.

3. **Answer:** A
   Rationale: Immobilization should be avoided. Ambulation prevents further bone resorption and hypercalcemia. Analgesics should be administered to relieve pain and help maintain mobility. B is incorrect; this action implies that adequate hydration prevents renal failure. C is incorrect because this precaution is appropriate to protect against pathologic fractures. D is incorrect; this action reflects the client's understanding regarding predisposition to hypercalcemia due to lytic bone lesions.

4. **Answer:** B
   Rationale: Option B is appropriate in the client's condition. Option A is incorrect. Options C and D are incorrect for this client.

5. **Answer:** D
   Rationale: Range of motion (ROM) is necessary to support ADL. Option A is incorrect; participation (B) by the client is not required. C may occur with all aging clients.

6. **Answer:** A
   Rationale: A change in position is correct; options B and C are useful. The client must change position frequently to decrease stasis, increase circulation, and decrease pressure in the area. Option D may be included in A.

7. **Answer:** C
   Rationale: There are no data to support the need for vital signs at this time. Baseline vital signs are appropriate for a client with an infection. Options A and B are appropriate in assessment of the client before carrying out the order. Option D is appropriate; if the client experiences pain, ROM exercise should be discontinued.

8. **Answer:** B
   Rationale: Reflective technique helps build a trusting nurse-client relationship because the client can express painful or uncomfortable feelings that are empathetically received by the nurse. Options A and D are incorrect because they contribute to the problem. Option C is incorrect; it does not show understanding of Mrs. G.'s behavior.

9. **Answer:** D
   Rationale: Options A, B, and C are reasonable expected outcomes. However, the most important is option D; her source of anxiety may change, but new ways of coping would enable her to handle her anxiety.

10. **Answer:** C
    Rationale: A calm demeanor is required because anxiety is easily transmitted and exacerbated. Support is also important for the anxious client. Options A, B, and D do not contribute to a therapeutic relationship.

11. **Answer:** C
    Rationale: In the event of moist desquamation, the client must be evaluated by the physician for the appropriate clinical intervention before radiation therapy is continued.

12. **Answer:** D
    Rationale: The nurse should be as specific as possible when addressing a confused, disoriented client. The other choices are incorrect. In A and B, questions about the environment and the need to make choices may be too challenging and may decrease the client's self-esteem. Choice C provides irrelevant information.

13. **Answer:** B
    Rationale: Safety from falls is a priority for this client. Options A, C, and D may all be necessary but are not essential.

14. *Answer:* A

Rationale: Succeeding at a task may increase self-esteem and motivation. Option B may have a negative, regressive effect. Option C is not contraindicated but is not likely to promote motivation and self-esteem. Option D may increase the client's frustration if the task is beyond the client's ability.

15. *Answer:* C

Rationale: Adequate daily exercise increases the likelihood that a client with insomnia will sleep at night. Daily napping is in direct opposition to sleeping at night. Sedatives (B) can be habit forming and should be used only as a last resort. Tea (D) is a caffeinated drink and will contribute to wakefulness.

16. *Answer:* D

Rationale: Changing the environment, even occasionally, can increase confusion. Options A, B, and C would not be contraindicated in the case of a client with alterations in mental status.

17. *Answer:* C

Rationale: Self-care helps promote independence and increases self-esteem through good hygiene habits. Option B is impractical; it is unrealistic to expect the client to take care of all her hygiene needs. Option D would be dishonest, would not benefit the client, and would promote dependence on the staff.

18. *Answer:* C

Rationale: The activity of combing the hair puts the shoulder joint through its range of motion. The other options also should be encouraged, but the best answer is C.

19. *Answer:* A

Rationale: Deep breathing and coughing help to mobilize secretions and decrease the risk of atelectasis. Elastic stockings (B) decrease the risk for thrombophlebitis. Fluids (option D) would help to liquefy secretions, but 1,500 mL may be insufficient. A semisitting position (C) may be appropriate, but without coughing this measure would be ineffective.

20. *Answer:* D

Rationale: Axillary lymph nodes are usually removed with a radical mastectomy. To facilitate drainage from the arm on the affected side, the arm should be elevated on pillows with the client's hand higher than her elbow and her elbow higher than her shoulder. The other options do not facilitate drainage from the arm.

21. *Answer:* C

Rationale: Redness is the most common reaction noted. Options A, B, and D are not commonly observed.

22. *Answer:* C

Rationale: Trochanter rolls alongside the legs from the ilium to midthigh will prevent external rotation of the hips. With option A, a firm pillow has been used to support the legs properly, but pillows should be used as a temporary measure as they do not hold the leg and hips in proper alignment over a period of time. Sandbags (B) do not effectively support the hips in proper alignment. A footboard (D) does not keep the legs and hips in proper body alignment for the client on bed rest.

23. *Answer:* B

Rationale: There is minimal pressure on the knee with respect to positioning. Areas of high pressure and remaining in positions for prolonged periods promote the development of decubitus ulcers.

24. *Answer:* A

Rationale: A helpless client should be positioned on his or her side, not the back. This position help secretions escape from the throat and mouth and minimizes the risk of aspiration. Options B, C, and D are all appropriate; suction equipment should be available; the client's mouth can be opened with a padded tongue blade, and the teeth should be cleaned with a toothbrush.

25. *Answer:* C

Rationale: The initial reaction when pressure is applied to the skin is that the area becomes blanched or whitish. Option A is incorrect; it relates to inadequate oxygen in the blood circulating in the area. Option B is incorrect; this is not the initial observation. Hyperemia or reddish skin occurs when pressure is relieved and the body then carries excess amounts of blood to the area to make up for the temporary depletion of blood supply. Option D is incorrect, as this observation is noted in skin because of hyperbilirubinemia and deposits of bile pigments as noted in someone with a disorder of the gallbladder or liver.

26. *Answer:* D
Rationale: The client is not deaf or hard of hearing; speaking louder is of little value. Options A, B, and C are appropriate techniques to use when communicating with an aphasic client.

27. *Answer:* D
Rationale: Providing positive reinforcement with patience as the client is making progress in his efforts to overcome impairments is a supportive intervention. Options A, B, and C have little supportive value.

28. *Answer:* A
Rationale: Options B, C, and D are all adversely affected by inactivity. Storage of vitamin B_{12} is the least influenced by activity.

29. *Answer:* D
Rationale: Phosphorus and calcium are important constituents of bone. Inactivity causes demineralization. Determination of serum levels would be most beneficial. Synovial fluid analysis (option A) is indicated for an inflammatory disease process. Option B is indicated for bony metastasis. Option C is indicated for an inflammatory process or infection and complaints of fatigue.

30. *Answer:* B
Rationale: A diet without fiber leaves little residual, and there is little mechanical stimulus for peristalsis. Options A, C, and D increase the risk for constipation.

31. *Answer:* A
Rationale: Lymphedema is more likely to occur when the limb is dependent. Keeping the arm above the level of the heart will help prevent lymphedema. Options B and C only decrease mobility. Option D is incorrect; it is potentially dangerous to apply heat to the arm.

32. *Answer:* D
Rationale: Washing her face requires movement from the elbow down without moving the shoulder at the axilla. Options A, B, and C all require movement of the shoulder.

33. *Answer:* D
Rationale: There is a 25% risk for the development of breast cancer in the contralateral breast. Option A is partially correct. Option B is inaccurate. Option C is also inaccurate; no woman should depend on the physician for breast examination.

34. *Answer:* A
Rationale: Because of a history of smoking, airway limitation in the lung tissue and structure has been chronic. Option D is incorrect; there is increased residual volume. Options B and C are both reduced.

35. *Answer:* C
Rationale: Strengthening the upper extremities will help Mrs. M. manipulate assistive devices postoperatively. Upper extremity strength is also needed to compensate for the changed center of gravity that occurs when a lower limb is lost. Options A, B, and D will not help or are potentially detrimental.

36. *Answer:* D
Rationale: Wrapping the stump with an elastic bandage in a figure-8 style helps to control edema and maintain the stump in a tapered shape that can more easily be fitted for a prosthesis. Options A, B, and C are not priorities in this situation.

37. *Answer:* A
Rationale: Foods high in sugar or acid content should be avoided. Options B and C will have a drying effect on the oral mucosa. Option D is an option but not for this situation.

38. *Answer:* B
Rationale: Hypercalcemia leads to release of calcium salts, which cause itching. Option A is incorrect. Anticholinergics are used as a smooth muscle relaxant. Antihistamines (C) are used in the treatment of allergic responses. Option D (promotion of hydration) is a treatment measure to decrease the discomfort of pruritus.

39. *Answer:* D
Rationale: Water-based lubricants promote hydration of the skin. Option A will promote drying of the skin, which may increase itching. Option B is incorrect; petroleum-based lubri-

cants clog the pores and prevent excretion and perspiration and increase the risk of pruritus. Option C promotes impaired skin integrity.

40. *Answer:* D
   Rationale: White patches are usually indicative of a fungal infectious process and can be serious if not treated. Option A should be done daily to detect the problem early. Option B is incorrect. White patches should never be removed. Option C is incorrect; diet will not prevent stomatitis.

41. *Answer:* C
   Rationale: This is the least abrasive and most effective regimen. Oral care should be done routinely. It involves no abrasive or drying agents that could promote stomatitis. Option A is incorrect. It contains an abrasive agent. Option B is incorrect. It contains a drying agent. Option D (commercial mouth washes) contains alcohol, which is a drying agent.

42. *Answer:* C
   Rationale: Both of these interventions aid in decreasing serum calcium. Option A does not promote calcium excretion. Options B and C (limiting mobility and fluid intake) are contraindicated.

43. *Answer:* C
   Rationale: It does not address the effects of hypercalcemia. Option A addresses mental status changes that can occur. Option B addresses the issues of itching, and D, the risk of fractures that can occur.

44. *Answer:* C
   Rationale: Changes in mental status are initial symptoms of hypercalcemia. Other assessments (options A, B, and D) indicate later changes.

45. *Answer:* C
   Rationale: Ensure safety for the client since weakness and confusion may be present. The client may not be aware of the need for assistance (option A). Options B and D are appropriate interventions but not critical to safe care in this situation.

46. *Answer:* C
   Rationale: Hepatic toxicity can cause delirium. It is characterized by jaundice, ascites, and changes in behavior. Options A, B, and D are incorrect.

47. *Answer:* B
   Rationale: Withdrawal is not an early sign of delirium. Options A, C, and D are all associated with delirium.

48. *Answer:* B
   Rationale: Social isolation has an adverse effect on the appetite. Options A, C, and D have a positive effect on the appetite.

49. *Answer:* B
   Rationale: The purpose is to build self-esteem and provide the client with some control. Option A may secure the client's cooperation and support, and option C may occur secondary to option B. D may also occur, but it is not a priority in this situation.

50. *Answer:* C
   Rationale: Self-administration of medications increases the risk of injury to the client. Insomnia (option A) and fatigue (option B) may aggravate the condition. Option D provides reassurance when the client is aware of the lack of control.

51. *Answer:* B
   Rationale: Pretreatment education may reduce client and family's anxiety and provide needed information to plan and adjust lifestyle and daily activities. Options A and D are inappropriate. Teaching is an essential part of the nurse's responsibility. Option C is inappropriate. Prevention and early detection are priorities in reversing many of the neurotoxicities.

52. *Answer:* C
   Rationale: The cerebellum is responsible for coordination and balance. Option A is for general CNS response, B assesses increased intraocular pressure, and D examines facial and hypoglossal nerves.

53. *Answer:* C
   Rationale: High cumulative doses can lead to long-term neuropathies of the hands and feet. Options A, B, and D are all incorrect.

54. *Answer:* D

Rationale: Phenytoin chloride is a neurologic medication used in the treatment of neuropathic pain. Options A, B, and C are all nonpharmacologic measures used to relieve pain.

55. *Answer:* B

Rationale: Restriction is not helpful, a social network is essential for adapting to the limitations of the disease. Option A provides environmental cues that are helpful in managing cognitive dysfunction. Option C provides a reminder and minimizes frustration. Option D provides some consistency and routine for activities.

BIBLIOGRAPHY

Baird, S.B., McCorkle, R., & Grant, M. (1996). Alterations in mobility. In S.B. Baird, R. McCorkle, & M. Grant (eds.). *Cancer Nursing: A Comprehensive Textbook.* Philadelphia: WB Saunders, pp. 850–863.

Bender, C. (1994). Cognitive dysfunction associated with biological response modifier therapy. *Oncol Nurs Forum 21*(3), 515–523.

Itano, J., & Taoka, K. (eds.). (1998). *Core Curriculum for Oncology Nursing* (3rd ed.). Philadelphia: WB Saunders.

Furlong, G.T. (1993). Neurologic complications of immunosuppressive cancer therapy. *Oncol Nurs Forum 20*(9), 1337–1354.

Groenwald, S., Frogge, M.H., Goodman, M., & Yarbro, C.H. (eds.). (1997). Late effects of cancer treatment. *Cancer Nursing: Principles and Practice* (4th ed.). Boston: Jones & Bartlett, pp. 669–679.

Ignatavicius, D.D., Workman, L., & Mishler, M.A. (1995). Problems of mobility, sensation, and cognition: Management of clients with problems of the nervous system. *Medical-Surgical Nursing: A Nursing Process Approach* (2nd ed.). Philadelphia: WB Saunders, pp. 1083–1293.

NOTES

12

Myelosuppression

Dawn Camp-Sorrell

Select the best answer for each of the following questions:

1. The immune system of a client with cancer may be depressed because of all the following *except*
   A. nutritional status.
   B. age.
   C. type of malignancy.
   D. continuous narcotic drip.

2. Granulocytes collectively include
   A. neutrophils, basophils, and eosinophils.
   B. neutrophils, lymphocytes, and basophils.
   C. monocytes, lymphocytes, and eosinophils.
   D. lymphocytes, neutrophils, and basophils.

3. Ms Brown presents to the clinic for her fourth course of chemotherapy for breast cancer. The absolute neutrophil count (ANC) is 1000/mm³. What would be the next step?
   A. Proceed with planned chemotherapy.
   B. Admit Ms Brown to the hospital for hydration.
   C. Begin antibiotics immediately.
   D. Teach Ms Brown infection precautions and what symptoms should prompt her to call the physician or nurse.

4. Which measure would be important to follow for a client with an ANC less than 500/mm³?
   A. Take a rectal temperature regularly.
   B. Administer broad-spectrum antibiotics if fever is present.
   C. Send fresh flowers to the room.
   D. Avoid bathing for 2 days.

5. During the nadir period from chemotherapy the client should be instructed to avoid all drugs that inhibit platelet function. Such drugs include
   A. aspirin.
   B. ibuprofen.
   C. indomethacin.
   D. all of the above.

6. Clients are at a severe risk of infection when the
   A. hemoglobin value is less than 10 g/dL.
   B. platelet count is less than 20,000/mm³.
   C. ANC is less than 1500/mm³.
   D. ANC is less than 500/mm³.

7. Clients are at a severe risk of bleeding when
   A. neutrophils are 50%.
   B. lymphocytes are 30%.
   C. platelets are less than 20,000.
   D. basophils are 0.

8. Mr. H. returns to the clinic to receive his sixth course of etoposide and cisplatin for small cell lung cancer. After obtaining his blood counts, the platelet level is reported to be 30,000. What would be your next step?
   A. Administer platelets immediately.
   B. Teach Mr. H. about bleeding precautions and what symptoms should prompt him to seek medical attention.
   C. Proceed with chemotherapy.
   D. Call hospice for placement.

9. Nadir is a term used to describe
   A. the highest point the WBCs reach after cancer treatment.

B. WBC lysis related to chemotherapy administration.

C. DNA content of the WBC.

D. the lowest point blood cells reach after a cancer treatment.

10. What is a major concern when administering amphotericin B?

A. Diarrhea.

B. Myelosuppression.

C. Fever and chills.

D. Hypersensitivity rash.

11. Ms Z. arrives at the hospital emergency department with fever, chills, and malaise. Her signs and symptoms are indicative of

A. anemia.

B. thrombocytopenia.

C. superior vena cava syndrome.

D. infection secondary to neutropenia.

12. When implementing a teaching plan for the client with a low ANC, the nurse should plan to do the following *except*

A. ensure privacy and freedom from interruptions.

B. include all family members in the discussion.

C. have written materials available for the client to keep.

D. initiate teaching when the client is in pain.

13. The client should be instructed to contact the physician immediately if which of the following side effects occurs?

A. Nosebleed that will not stop after applying pressure.

B. Temperature of 99.6° F.

C. One episode of nausea without vomiting after chemotherapy.

D. Body hair begins to fall out after chemotherapy.

14. Which of the following drugs can produce a fever?

A. Interferon, methotrexate, adriamycin.

B. Interferon, interleukin, vancomycin.

C. Interleukin-2, penicillin, amphotericin B.

D. Tumor necrosis factor, gentamycin, vancomycin.

15. Mr. S. presents to the clinic with a temperature of 102° F. What initial question would you

ask in taking his history to determine risk for infection?

A. Have you recently been treated for your cancer with chemotherapy, radiation, or biotherapy?

B. Have you recently been outside the United States?

C. Are you still taking your coumadin every day?

D. Have you been experiencing dizziness, fatigue, or shortness of breath?

16. Ms Walters returns for her next chemotherapy treatment; however, her ANC is 1300. Which cells of the WBC differential will predict the recovery of neutrophils?

A. Eosinophils.

B. Monocytes.

C. Basophils.

D. Neutrophils.

17. Myelosuppression is defined as the reduction in bone marrow function that results in a reduced release of which cells into the peripheral circulation?

A. Red blood cells, megakarocytes, and tumor necrosis factor.

B. Red blood cells, white blood cells, and platelets.

C. White blood cells, erythroblasts, and colony-stimulating factors.

D. Platelets, red blood cells, and interleukin.

18. Neutropenia describes a decrease in the number of circulating

A. basophils.

B. white blood cells.

C. neutrophils.

D. red blood cells.

19. Neutrophils are the first line of the body's defense against

A. destroying viruses that invade the body.

B. destroying bacterial infection.

C. destroying fungal infection.

D. destroying parasites.

20. Clients who are at high risk for becoming neutropenic include all *except*

A. older clients who have more fat and less cellular marrow.

B. clients with tumor invasion of the bone marrow.

MYELOSUPPRESSION • QUESTIONS **73**

C. clients with a high negative nitrogen balance.

D. clients who received radiation to the lower left calf for sarcoma.

21. Radiation to which of the following areas can result in myelosuppression?
    A. Ilia, vertebrae, ribs, skull, sternum, and long bones.
    B. Tibia, ribs, skull, and sternum.
    C. Ulna, sternum, and vertebrae.
    D. Skull, ribs, patella, and metacarpals.

22. The nurse should recognize that steroids will mask the occurrence of an infection by
    A. competing at the complement site with tumor necrosis factor.
    B. decreasing the production of B cells.
    C. preventing the migration of neutrophils to the bacteria.
    D. preventing the antigen and antibody reaction.

23. Antiviral medications are usually administered to the febrile neutropenic client when
    A. the absolute neutrophil count is less than 500/mm^3.
    B. the fever continues for 3 days after antibiotics are initiated.
    C. the client has undergone high-dose chemotherapy.
    D. mucosal lesions or viral disease is suspected.

24. Hematopoietic growth factors are administered to
    A. prevent neutropenia.
    B. prevent anemia.
    C. promote proliferation and differentiation of progenitor cells along multiple cell pathways.
    D. promote the proliferation and differentiation of interleukin.

25. Growth factors for neutrophils are usually initiated *except when*
    A. a client is at high risk for febrile neutropenia from high-dose chemotherapy.
    B. a client undergoes an autologous bone marrow transplant.

C. a client experienced a previous febrile neutropenic episode with chemotherapy administration.

D. chemotherapy dose is reduced.

26. When the client's nadir persists for more than 7 to 10 days, the risk increases for
    A. severe infection.
    B. compromised myelosuppression.
    C. resistant organisms to treatment.
    D. severe blood clots.

27. As the neutrophils decrease, the only sign of infection may be
    A. purulent drainage from a vascular access device.
    B. petechiae on the lower extremities.
    C. fever.
    D. dry hacking cough.

28. The best measure to institute to prevent infection in the client with low absolute neutrophil count is
    A. encourage visitors.
    B. encourage the client to bathe every 2 days.
    C. strict handwashing.
    D. use of a laminar flow room.

29. Thrombocytopenia describes
    A. a decrease in the circulating platelets below 100,000/mm^3.
    B. a decrease in the circulating white blood cells below 1500/mm^3.
    C. a decrease in the circulating neutrophils below 1000/mm^3.
    D. a decrease in the circulating red blood cells below 1000/mm^3.

30. Clients at high risk for developing thrombocytopenia include all *except* those experiencing
    A. hypocoagulation disorders such as liver disease or vitamin K deficiency.
    B. hypercoagulation disorders such as paraneoplastic syndromes.
    C. high doses of interferon.
    D. high doses of vinblastine.

31. After chemotherapy administration, the platelet count usually decreases
    A. before the white blood cells decrease.
    B. in 7 to 14 days after the administration of chemotherapy.

C. after the red blood cells decrease.

D. in 28 days after chemotherapy administration.

32. Some medications that can alter platelet function are
    A. aspirin, digitalis, and digoxin.
    B. milk of magnesia, heparin, and quinidine.
    C. Senokot, furosemide, and phenytoin.
    D. acetaminophen, sulfonamides, and penicillin.

33. The method(s) for transmitting infectious organisms to clients include
    A. direct contact.
    B. indirect contact.
    C. airborne transmission.
    D. all of the above.

34. Risk factors for infection include all *except*
    A. altered mucosal barriers.
    B. trimming finger and toe nails.
    C. recent exposure to an infectious organism.
    D. receiving multimodal treatment.

35. If the client is at high risk for infection, measures that can be initiated to minimize the occurrence are
    A. inserting a urinary catheter to monitor the urine output.
    B. leaving all wounds open to air.
    C. encouraging daily personal hygiene, oral hygiene, and perineal care.
    D. flushing all lumens of a long-term catheter every 8 hours.

36. Hemorrhage describes the occurrence of
    A. platelet count less than 50,000/mm³.
    B. red blood cell count less than 100,000/mm³.
    C. abnormal internal or external discharge of blood.
    D. fibrinogen level less than 30 mL.

37. Hemorrhage can result from all *except*
    A. brain metastases.
    B. myeloproliferative disorders.

C. a vascular access device with a fibrin sheath.

D. disseminated intravascular coagulation.

38. Consequence of prolonged hemorrhage include
    A. shock.
    B. increase in fluid volume.
    C. decrease in circulating cancer cells.
    D. increase in cardiac output.

39. Fever can result from
    A. infection.
    B. administration of certain drugs such as vancomycin.
    C. biotherapy agents.
    D. all the above.

40. Clients who experience the following are at a high risk for fever *except* those who
    A. have central nervous system and hepatic metastasis.
    B. are 2 weeks postoperative.
    C. have an absolute neutrophil count less than 500/mm³.
    D. are receiving interferon therapy.

41. Ms C. calls the clinic and reports a fever of 101° F for the past 24 hours. This fever would not be uncommon if the client received any of the following *except*
    A. bleomycin administration.
    B. biotherapy administration.
    C. vancomycin.
    D. indomethacin for bone metastasis pain.

42. Prolonged fever and chills experienced by the client can lead to
    A. increase in fatigue.
    B. decrease in circulating cancer cells.
    C. increase in activity.
    D. decrease in the occurrence of infection.

43. Comfort measures that should be instituted when the client is experiencing a fever include all *except*
    A. reducing the amount of clothing worn by the patient.
    B. providing tepid sponge baths.
    C. changing damp clothing immediately.
    D. avoiding the use of acetaminophen.

ANSWERS

1. *Answer:* D
Rationale: Answers A, B, and C can depress the client's immune system. Narcotics do not interfere with the immune system.

2. *Answer:* A
Rationale: Answer A lists the cells referred to as granulocytes.

3. *Answer:* D
Rationale: Response A is incorrect because most physicians do not administer chemotherapy if the ANC is less than 1500/mm^3 or WBC less than 1000/mm^3. B and C are incorrect because the patient does not have a fever or signs of dehydration. D is the correct response to teach Ms Brown what measures to take to prevent infection and when to call for medical assistance. A WBC could reflect Ms Brown's immune system's ability to fight infection, but an ANC is more reflective since the neutrophils can be low when the WBC is normal.

4. *Answer:* B
Rationale: Answers A, C, and D are not appropriate infection precautions. Broad-spectrum antibiotics should be administered when fever is present to prevent further untoward effects of the infection such as sepsis.

5. *Answer:* D
Rationale: Answers A, B, and C are correct. Each of these drugs has the tendency to inhibit platelet function.

6. *Answer:* D
Rationale: Answer A refers to anemia; B refers to thrombocytopenia; C the ANC is not low. Answer D is correct. The lower the ANC below 1000/mm^3, the higher the risk for infection.

7. *Answer:* C
Rationale: Answers A, B, and D refer to the white blood cells. Answer C is correct because levels of platelets below 20,000 increase the client's risk for severe bleeding.

8. *Answer:* B
Rationale: Answer A is incorrect. Unless the client is actively bleeding, platelets are usually administered for levels of 20,000 or lower. Answer C is incorrect. Chemotherapy is usually held if the platelet count is less than 100,000. Answer D is incorrect. Answer B is correct because the client is at risk for spontaneous bleeding and should follow bleeding precautions.

9. *Answer:* D
Rationale: Answers A, B, and C do not give the correct definition of nadir. Nadir refers to the lowest point.

10. *Answer:* C
Rationale: Amphotericin B can cause fever and chills during administration.

11. *Answer:* D
Rationale: These are signs of infection.

12. *Answer:* D
Rationale: Learning cannot be accomplished if the client is experiencing pain.

13. *Answer:* A
Rationale: A nosebleed that is difficult to control should alert the nurse that the client may have a low platelet count.

14. *Answer:* B
Rationale: All of these drugs can induce fever.

15. *Answer:* A
Rationale: This information would provide the nurse with the approximate time to expect the client's nadir and to suspect an infection with the presentation of a fever.

16. *Answer:* B
Rationale: The monocyte count is usually elevated before the neutrophils recover.

17. *Answer:* B
Rationale: Red blood cells, white blood cells, and platelets are mature cells that are released into the peripheral circulation from the bone marrow.

18. *Answer:* C
Rationale: A decrease in neutrophils in the blood is referred to neutropenia.

19. *Answer:* B
Rationale: Neutrophils provide the first line of the body's defense against bacterial infection by localizing and neutralizing bacteria.

20. *Answer:* D
Rationale: Clients who receive radiation to a major bone marrow production site such as the sternum, skull, pelvic or long bones will be at risk for becoming neutropenic with subsequent treatments, as are clients with hematologic malignancies or blood dyscrasia.

21. *Answer:* A
Rationale: Radiation of 20 Gy or more to the major bone marrow production sites will result in myelosuppression.

22. *Answer:* C
Rationale: Steroids prevent migration of neutrophils to the bacteria and the process of phagocytosis.

23. *Answer:* D
Rationale: Antiviral drugs are usually not initiated unless the client is undergoing a bone marrow transplant or the client exhibits signs of a virus such as an oral lesion.

24. *Answer:* C
Rationale: Hematopoietic growth factors promote the proliferation and differentiation of hematopoietic progenitor cells along multiple pathways. Growth factors do not prevent neutropenia or anemia but promote production of the cells in anemic or neutropenic clients.

25. *Answer:* D
Rationale: If the chemotherapy dose is reduced and will not compromise the goal of cancer treatment, growth factor is not recommended. However, if the dose cannot be reduced, growth factor would be prescribed.

26. *Answer:* A
Rationale: When the client experiences a prolonged nadir, the risk for severe infection increases.

27. *Answer:* C
Rationale: Fever may be the only response to an infection because of the inhibition of phago-cytic cells; therefore, erythema, inflammation, and drainage may be minimal or absent.

28. *Answer:* C
Rationale: Strict handwashing will prevent up to 90% of exogenous organisms that come in direct contact with the client.

29. *Answer:* A
Rationale: When platelet levels drop below 100,000/mm^3, the client has thrombocytopenia.

30. *Answer:* C
Rationale: Although the biotherapeutic agents modulate the immune system, the potential for alteration of the blood cells remains unknown. The occurrence of thrombocytopenia after high doses of interferon has not been evident in clinical studies.

31. *Answer:* B
Rationale: Platelet counts usually decrease in 7 to 14 days after administration of chemotherapy after the decrease in white blood cells.

32. *Answer:* A
Rationale: All these drugs can alter platelet function.

33. *Answer:* D
Rationale: Each method can transmit organisms to the client. The most common method is direct contact.

34. *Answer:* B
Rationale: Trimming nails helps prevent infectious organisms from colonizing such as fungus.

35. *Answer:* C
Rationale: Promoting meticulous hygiene can minimize the occurrence of organisms colonizing.

36. *Answer:* C
Rationale: Hemorrhage is the result of abnormal internal or external bleeding.

37. *Answer:* C
Rationale: Hemorrhage does not occur from a clot that is formed on a device.

38. *Answer:* A
   Rationale: Shock will occur with a decrease in fluid volume, which will result in decreased cardiac output and decreased tissue perfusion.

39. *Answer:* D
   Rationale: All of these factors can cause fever.

40. *Answer:* B
   Rationale: Clients who are 2 weeks from an operative procedure are unlikely to experience a fever.

41. *Answer:* D
   Rationale: Indomethacin is often given to reduce tumor-induced fever.

42. *Answer:* A
   Rationale: Prolonged fever and chills results in an increase in metabolic activity and oxygen consumption, which lead to an increase of fatigue.

43. *Answer:* D
   Rationale: Acetaminophen alternated with aspirin and nonsteroidal antiinflammatory drugs if not contraindicated can be administered every 4 hours to decrease fever.

BIBLIOGRAPHY

Camp-Sorrell, D. (1996). Hematologic toxicities. In M. Liebman & D. Camp-Sorrell (eds.). *Multimodal Therapy in Oncology Nursing.* St. Louis: Mosby, pp. 367–385.

Finkbine, K.L., & Ernst, T.F. (1993). Drug therapy management of the febrile neutropenic cancer patient. *Canc Prac 1,* 295–304.

Friedberg, R.C. (1994). Issues in transfusion therapy in the patient with malignancy. *Hematol Oncol Clin North Am 8*(6), 1223–1253.

Giamarellou, H. (1995). Empiric therapy for infections in the febrile, neutropenic, compromised host. *Med Clin North Am 79*(3), 559–580.

Miller, L.L., Anderson, J.R., Anderson, P.N., et al. (1994). American Society of Clinical Oncology recommendations for the use of hematopoietic colony-stimulating factors: Evidence-based clinical practice guidelines. *J Clin Oncol 12,* 2471–2508.

Shuey, K.M. (1996). Platelet-associated bleeding disorders. *Semin Oncol Nurs 12*(1), 15–27.

NOTES

PART III

Gastrointestinal and Urinary Function

13

Alterations in Nutrition

April J. Dumond and Robi Thomas

Select the best answer for each of the following questions:

1. Which would *not* be a key assessment factor of a client with xerostomia?
   A. Overall status of teeth and gums.
   B. Impact of xerostomia on daily life.
   C. Status of mucous membranes.
   D. Pattern of elimination.

2. After receiving radiation therapy to the head and neck for 1 week, a client reports difficulty chewing, swallowing, and speaking. He has no appetite. His oral mucous membranes are dry, and his saliva is thick and scanty. He denies pain. He most likely has
   A. stomatitis.
   B. herpes simplex.
   C. buccal inflammation.
   D. xerostomia.

3. Mr. J. is to begin radiation therapy to a field that includes the salivary glands. Which of the following factors would increase the risk of xerostomia?
   A. Alcohol ingestion.
   B. Digitalis preparations.
   C. Poor dentition.
   D. Steroid therapy.

4. Which of the following agents is used to reduce the severity of xerostomia and salivary dysfunction by stimulating remaining salivary gland function?
   A. Viscous lidocaine.
   B. Ondansetron.
   C. Pilocarpine.
   D. Sucralfate.

5. Mrs. H. is a 68-year-old client with metastatic head and neck cancer; she has had radical neck dissection, radiation therapy, and chemotherapy. She tells the hospice nurse that her mouth is dry and that it interferes with eating and swallowing. Which of the following statements indicate that Mrs. H. understands her condition and how to treat it?
   A. I should try eating spicy foods and citrus juices that may help me produce more saliva.
   B. I need to drink 8 glasses of liquids per day.
   C. I need to be sure to wear my false teeth most of the time, even though they don't fit very well.
   D. I should avoid ice chips and popsicles, since they can damage my remaining salivary glands.

6. Which of the following is *not* a complication of xerostomia that would require medical intervention?
   A. Weight loss over 10 pounds.
   B. Aspirational pneumonia.
   C. Infection in the oral cavity.
   D. Lesions or ulcerations of the oral cavity.

7. Which of the following regimens would you recommend to a client at risk for developing stomatitis?
   A. Schedule oral care q2h with a soft toothbrush and nonfluoridated abrasive dentifrice to remove debris.

B. Rinse mouth q2h while awake and q4h during the night with a baking soda and peroxide rinse.

C. Schedule oral care q2–4h while awake with a soft toothbrush, fluoridated toothpaste, and oral irrigations of baking soda, salt, and water.

D. Continue with current oral care—twice-a-day brushing and rinse with commercial rinses—until stomatitis actually develops.

8. In teaching Ms S. about her continuous fluorouracil infusion, the nurse includes instructions about the importance of an oral care protocol. These instructions include

A. performing an assessment of the oral cavity on a weekly basis.

B. removing white patches gently if present on the tongue or mouth and applying a lanolin-based gel.

C. beginning a low-residue, semisoft diet to prevent stomatitis.

D. calling the doctor immediately if white patches appear on the tongue or mouth.

9. Which of the following chemotherapy agents has a greater risk for causing stomatitis?

A. 5-Fluorouracil.

B. Dacarbazine.

C. Cisplatin.

D. Vinblastine.

10. Mucositis is defined as

A. inflammatory response of mucosal cells of the oral cavity.

B. inflammatory response of mucosal cells of the esophagus.

C. inflammatory response of mucosal cells of the intestine.

D. inflammatory response of mucosal cells of the entire gastrointestinal tract, from mouth to rectum.

11. Which client is at greatest risk for mucositis of the oral cavity?

A. Client with lung cancer, receiving radiation therapy.

B. Client with leukemia, undergoing bone marrow transplantation.

C. Client with colorectal cancer, after colon resection.

D. Client with glioblastoma multiforme, after craniotomy.

12. M., an 11-year-old boy with non-Hodgkin's lymphoma, has completed CHOP therapy and has just returned to school. He presents to the school nurse with a complaint of a sore mouth. On inspection, the nurse notes erythema of the oral mucosa with isolated small white patches and ulcerations on the palate. M.'s temperature is 99.6° F. After consulting with the oncology nurse in the pediatric oncology clinic, the school nurse calls M.'s mother. Which of the following statements indicates that M.'s mother understands how to care for M. and manage his symptoms?

A. I need to be sure that M. brushes his teeth at least twice a day and eats a lot of popsicles.

B. I don't need to take him to the doctor unless his mouth starts to bleed or his temperature goes over 101° F.

C. M. has stomatitis and needs frequent, careful mouth care. He also needs to see his doctor, since the white patches may mean that he has an infection.

D. M. needs to take steroids to clear up his mouth sores.

13. Which of the following is *not* an important factor to consider in the assessment of taste alterations in persons with cancer?

A. Taste alterations can lead to anorexia.

B. Taste alterations can lead to positive nitrogen balance.

C. Taste alterations can indicate stomatitis.

D. Taste alterations can indicate disease progression.

14. Mrs. B. is worried about her husband's nutrition. Since starting chemotherapy, he states, "Nothing tastes right." What advice would you give Mrs. B.?

A. Continue to prepare meals as usual. Eventually his taste will return to normal (about 2 weeks after therapy).

B. There is nothing you can do; this happens to everyone on chemotherapy.

C. Try to increase his intake of meat because it is a good source of protein and is generally well tolerated.

D. Try to increase sensitivity of taste buds by using spices and herbs in meal preparation.

15. A common taste alteration is a

A. decreased threshold for sweets.

B. craving for red meats.

C. sweet taste in the mouth.

D. decreased threshold for bitter tastes.

16. Which of the following interventions is *not* appropriate for managing taste alterations?

A. Use commercial mouthwashes, such as Scope or Listerine, to eliminate the bacteria that cause bad tastes.

B. Continue diligent oral care and inspection of the mucosa to ensure early identification of complications like infections.

C. Suggest that the client try meats served cold (such as turkey or ham), as they are usually better tolerated and have less of a metallic taste.

D. Have the client suck on sugarfree lemon drops or other smooth, flat tart candies to stimulate saliva.

17. A decrease in the acuity of the taste sensation is called

A. ageusia.

B. dysgeusia.

C. hypogeusia.

D. sialagogue.

18. A common infection *most likely* to cause taste alterations is

A. bacterial pneumonia.

B. oral candidiasis.

C. herpes zoster.

D. gram-positive infection of the oral cavity.

19. Ms L. timidly informs you that every time she comes to the clinic for chemotherapy she begins to feel nauseated, even before she gets her treatment. She cannot understand why this happens. Your response is

A. Don't worry about it. It happens to everyone.

B. What you are feeling is anticipatory nausea. It is a conditioned response some people experience with chemotherapy.

C. Try to eat before coming to the clinic. This will decrease that queasy feeling.

D. Do not eat after 12 AM the night before your clinic appointment. This will decrease your chance of vomiting.

20. All of the following interventions help to relieve nausea *except*

A. medicating with an antiemetic each time vomiting is experienced.

B. avoiding fatty or spicy foods.

C. medicating with an antiemetic on a round-the-clock basis until nausea subsides.

D. using relaxation or visual imagery techniques.

21. Which of the following settings may help to reduce nausea for a client receiving chemotherapy?

A. A bright, sunny, warm room to avoid chilling and depression.

B. A large treatment room with many other patients to distract the client.

C. A busy treatment area near the nurses' lounge to keep the client from feeling lonely.

D. A quiet, darkened, cool area, free of noise, noxious smells, and sights.

22. Which of these clients would be *most likely* to experience nausea related to chemotherapy?

A. 30-year-old woman, mother of two, who experienced severe "morning sickness" throughout her entire pregnancies.

B. 60-year-old man who had motion sickness as a child.

C. 48-year-old male alcoholic.

D. 20-year-old woman with no significant history of emesis.

23. Potential causes of nausea are

A. obstruction of a portion of the gastrointestinal tract or delayed gastric emptying.

B. stimulation of the true vomiting center (TVC) or the chemoreceptor trigger zone (CTZ).

C. increased intracranial pressure from a primary or metastatic central nervous system lesion.

D. all of the above.

24. Ms L. has non-Hodgkin's lymphoma. She experiences severe nausea with every chemotherapy treatment, and the nausea continues for up to 2 weeks after each treatment. Which statement by Ms L. indicates that she needs further instruction on management of her nausea?

A. I need to call the doctor if I lose more than 10% of my body weight.

B. I should try bland, chilled foods, and I should drink liquids separately from my meals.

C. I need to lie down for an hour after each meal to prevent nausea.

D. I will discuss my nausea with my physician to see if a different antiemetic may provide better control of my nausea.

25. Which of the following drugs has the highest emetogenic potential?
    A. Cisplatin.
    B. Vinblastine.
    C. Etoposide.
    D. Bleomycin.

26. Prolonged vomiting can lead to
    A. fluid and electrolyte imbalances.
    B. anorexia and weight loss.
    C. refusal to complete treatment plan or noncompliance.
    D. all of the above.

27. Mr. N., a 27-year-old client with germ cell cancer, receives BEP (bleomycin, etoposide, and cisplatin) every 3 weeks. To manage his nausea and vomiting, he takes oral ondansetron (Zofran). Which statement indicates that Mr. N. understands management of his nausea and vomiting?
    A. Zofran may cause me to become constipated, so I should take stool softeners.
    B. I only need to take Zofran if I start vomiting.
    C. I should continue to take Zofran two or three times a day for about 10 days after my chemotherapy is finished to prevent further vomiting.
    D. Zofran may cause drowsiness and unusual symptoms called extrapyramidal reactions.

28. Mr. T., a 50-year-old client with melanoma, is receiving dacarbazine (DTIC) and interferon. He tells you that he has almost continuous nausea and frequent vomiting daily. He is taking Compazine suppositories PRN but usually only takes one or two suppositories a day. Mr. T. says that he was hesitant to inform the health care team of his symptoms because he did not want to be "a baby." What is the nurse's best response?
    A. You must be having a lot of anxiety and stress, or you would not be feeling so bad.
    B. There are a number of other things we can try to decrease your symptoms. Tell me more about how you are feeling.

C. Both of these drugs can cause prolonged nausea and vomiting. There's really nothing else we can do to manage it.

D. Take one suppository every time you vomit.

29. The following statements about use of corticosteroids in the management of vomiting are true *except*
    A. Corticosteroids work well in combination with other antiemetics to control vomiting from highly emetogenic chemotherapy drugs.
    B. Rapid intravenous administration of corticosteroids may cause transient perineal, perioral, or abdominal burning and itching.
    C. Beware of classic steroid side effects, even when used for a short time.
    D. When steroids are used for a short time, classic steroid side effects do not occur.

30. Mr. W., a 68-year-old terminally ill client with cancer of the pancreas, has intractable nausea and vomiting. His wife discusses this with the hospice nurse. Which statement indicates that Mrs. W. needs further instruction about Mr. W.'s care?
    A. Vomiting is common in terminal clients, especially ones with pancreatic cancer.
    B. Since Mr. W. can't keep down nausea pills, we should try rectal suppositories.
    C. If the suppositories aren't effective, a continuous infusion of Reglan or Haldol may work.
    D. We should give him something that will keep him asleep, so he won't vomit.

31. Which of the following is *not* a sequela of prolonged anorexia?
    A. Lean body mass depletion.
    B. Visceral mass depletion.
    C. Constipation.
    D. Decreased immune function.

32. Which of the following would not be used as an intervention to prevent or eliminate anorexia?
    A. Consume nutritionally dense foods throughout the day.
    B. Avoid foods that are gas forming.
    C. Encourage clients to eat high-calorie foods.
    D. Encourage clients to eat five servings of fruits and vegetables throughout the day.

33. Which of the following is *not* a sign or symptom of dehydration?
    A. Esophagitis.
    B. Decreased urinary output.
    C. Delayed wound healing.
    D. Poor skin turgor.

34. Which client would *not* necessarily be at risk for dysphagia?
    A. Client with head and neck cancer.
    B. Client with multiple myeloma.
    C. Elderly client.
    D. Client with lung cancer with lymph node involvement.

35. Which of the following would *not* be used as a thickening agent?
    A. Thick-It.
    B. Nutra-Thik.
    C. Thick 'N Easy.
    D. Sustacal.

36. Which of the following types of foods would *not* be recommended for a client who is experiencing dysphagia?
    A. Ice chips.
    B. Mexican food.
    C. Pureed food.
    D. Semisolid food.

37. Which is the correct definition of xerostomia?
    A. An increase of saliva in the oral cavity.
    B. Difficulty swallowing.
    C. Abnormal or excessive dryness of the mouth due to a decrease of saliva.
    D. An inflammatory response of the epithelial cells on the surface of the gastrointestinal tract.

38. Which of the following would *not* be a measure used to provide moisture to the oral mucosa?
    A. Encourage the client to eat foods that he or she likes.
    B. Encourage the client to eat food that has gravy or milk in it.
    C. Encourage the client to drink liquids with meals.
    D. Encourage the client to eat popsicles.

39. Which of the following is *not* a type of mucositis?
    A. Stomatitis.
    B. Esophagitis.

    C. Gingivitis.
    D. Enteritis.

40. Your client has received cisplatin and is now complaining of a metallic taste in her mouth. Which of the following would you assume the client was experiencing?
    A. Hypogeusia.
    B. Dysgeusia.
    C. Ageusia.
    D. Stomatitis.

41. Your client has had a bone marrow transplant and is about to be discharged from the hospital. You are doing discharge teaching, and your client states that she still has trouble eating because the food tastes different and asks you how long this will last. Which is the correct response?
    A. Not long—as soon as your blood counts return to normal, your taste buds will return.
    B. Within 3 months—it takes 100 days after chemotherapy for abnormal taste sensation to disappear.
    C. This can last for up to a year after therapy. Try a variety of foods to find which foods taste good to you.
    D. Unfortunately, the abnormal taste sensation may never completely disappear.

42. You are a radiation oncology nurse and you are doing some pretreatment teaching. Your client is to receive a total of 2 Gy of radiation to head and neck area. You tell the client that he can expect his taste buds to change at what time frame?
    A. Day 10 to 14 and will last for approximately 20 days.
    B. Day 21 and will last for approximately 10 days.
    C. Day 7 and will last for approximately 21 days.
    D. Day 28 and will last for 28 days.

43. Which of the following drugs is not known to commonly affect taste sensation?
    A. Cisplatin.
    B. Cyclophosphamide.
    C. Methotrexate.
    D. Paclitaxel.

44. You are doing some prechemotherapy teaching and are discussing mucositis. The most im-

portant reason for trying to prevent or control mucositis is
- A. comfort.
- B. infection.
- C. self-image or self-esteem.
- D. recurrence of the cancer.

45. Your client has received intravenous chemotherapy and is experiencing esophagitis. He asks you why this is happening, since he didn't swallow the chemotherapy drug. Your answer would include which of the following?
- A. You have esophageal cancer; the esophagitis is due to the tumor's dissolving.
- B. Chemotherapy affects all mucosal epithelial cells, which includes the cells in the gastrointestinal tract.
- C. The side effect of the chemotherapeutic agent you received is that it affects your esophagus.
- D. This is an unusual occurrence; let me call your physician.

46. Mrs. R. is concerned about her husband's difficulty in swallowing since he had radiation therapy. She calls you for advice about dietary modifications. You advise her to
- A. maintain the current diet but have her husband tilt his head back to allow the passage of food.
- B. provide soft or semisoft foods.
- C. provide only high-calorie, high-protein liquids to avoid choking.
- D. keep the client NPO until dysphagia subsides.

47. Two weeks ago Mr. S. completed radiation therapy to a field that included his esophagus. He complains of difficulty swallowing and a feeling that food gets "stuck." Which of the following could affect his dysphagia?
- A. Stomatitis.
- B. Tracheostomy.
- C. Dental caries.
- D. Leukopenia.

48. A referral to which team member would be suggested for management of unresolved swallowing problems?
- A. Respiratory therapist.
- B. Speech therapist.
- C. Physical therapist.
- D. Oral surgeon.

49. Which of the following would *not* be an appropriate nursing diagnosis for potential complications of dysphagia?
- A. Alteration in nutritional status.
- B. Alteration in fluid and electrolyte balance.
- C. Alteration in protective mechanisms.
- D. Alteration in safety related to potential for aspiration.

50. Mrs. J. has lymphoma. She has had a dramatic response to chemotherapy and is at risk for tumor lysis syndrome. Which of the following findings would cue the nurse to a significant electrolyte imbalance?
- A. Tachycardia.
- B. Constipation.
- C. Hypertension.
- D. Muscle cramps.

51. Mrs. S. has breast cancer with metastasis to the bone. She is at risk for hypercalcemia. Which of the following assessments would be the initial change indicating clinical symptoms of hypercalcemia?
- A. Respiratory rate.
- B. Muscle tone.
- C. Mental status.
- D. Urinary output.

52. Mr. K. is receiving amphotericin and is at risk for hypokalemia. Which assessment would be most important in clinically detecting hypokalemia?
- A. Blood pressure.
- B. Skin turgor.
- C. Deep tendon reflexes.
- D. Appetite.

53. Mr. P. has hypokalemia. In evaluating choices that he made on his dietary menu, which of the following choices would indicate a need for additional dietary teaching?
- A. Bananas.
- B. Potato chips.
- C. Gatorade.
- D. Apples.

54. Mrs. C. is being treated with high-volume saline solution infusions for hypercalcemia (Ca^{2+} = 14.5 mEq/L). Which of the following nursing interventions would be critical in providing safe care for Mrs. C.?

A. Encourage Mrs. C. to ask for help when ambulating to the bathroom.
B. Measure the urine output after every void.
C. Assist Mrs. C. to a bedside commode every 1 to 2 hours.
D. Clean and dry the perineum after each void.

55. Mr. B., an elderly man with lung cancer, presents to the emergency department with a 5-day history of vomiting. Physical examination reveals shallow, slow respirations, irregular pulse, and muscle twitching. He appears disoriented and irritable. Blood gas analysis reveals pH (plasma) of 7.4 and bicarbonate of 29 mEq/L. Mr. B. is experiencing which complication of prolonged vomiting?
A. Metabolic alkalosis.
B. Metabolic acidosis.
C. Hypernatremia.
D. Hypokalemia.

56. The most common cause of hypercalcemia among hospitalized clients is
A. thiazide diuretic therapy.
B. decreased prostaglandin production.
C. malignancies with bone metastases.
D. Paget's disease of the bone.

57. Hypercalcemia is a complication most often seen in which malignancy?
A. Breast cancer.
B. Leukemia.
C. Glioblastoma.
D. Chondrosarcoma.

58. Nursing care of the client with bone metastases and hypercalcemia should include increased mobilization and adequate hydration to avoid which of the following sequelae?
A. Skin breakdown with formation of decubiti.
B. Increased release of calcium from bone.
C. Susceptibility to infection such as pneumonia.
D. Loss of function with formation of contractures.

59. Signs and symptoms related to the syndrome of inappropriate antidiuretic hormone (SIADH) include all of the following *except*
A. serum hyponatremia.
B. constipation.
C. fluid retention.
D. headache.

60. Signs of cachexia include all of the following *except*
A. weight loss greater than 10% of ideal body weight.
B. tissue wasting.
C. anorexia.
D. nausea and vomiting.

61. The *most common* side effect of administering enteral feedings too rapidly is
A. constipation.
B. vomiting.
C. diarrhea.
D. alopecia.

ANSWERS

1. *Answer:* D
   Rationale: Xerostomia relates to conditions of the oral cavity.

2. *Answer:* D
   Rationale: Clients with xerostomia have dry mucous membranes and difficulty with oral intake. Pain is not a factor.

3. *Answer:* A
   Rationale: Alcohol use dries mucous membranes.

4. *Answer:* C
   Rationale: Pilocarpine, a systemic parasympathomimetic originally used in ophthalmic solutions, has been studied and used to reduce the severity of xerostomia. Viscous lidocaine and sucralfate are used for mucositis; ondansetron is an antiemetic.

5. *Answer:* B
   Rationale: Clients with xerostomia should increase oral fluid intake. Spicy and acidic foods may worsen symptoms. Poor-fitting dentures should not be worn. Ice chips and popsicles may help xerostomia symptoms.

6. *Answer:* B
   Rationale: Aspirational pneumonia is a complication of dysphagia, not xerostomia. The other responses are complications of xerostomia; all require medical intervention.

7. *Answer:* C
   Rationale: This is the least abrasive and most effective program. It is done routinely and contains no abrasive or drying agents that could promote stomatitis.

8. *Answer:* D
   Rationale: White patches indicate an infectious process (usually fungal) and can be serious if not treated. Oral assessment should be done at least once daily. White patches should never be removed. Diet will not prevent stomatitis.

9. *Answer:* A
   Rationale: 5-Fluorouracil is a chemotherapy drug associated with a high incidence of stomati-

tis. It interferes with the normal replacement of epithelial cells.

10. *Answer:* D
    Rationale: Mucositis is a general term that describes the inflammatory response of mucosal epithelial cells that are present on all surfaces of the gastrointestinal tract from the mouth to the rectum. Stomatitis is mucositis in the oral cavity. Esophagitis is mucositis in the esophagus. Enteritis is mucositis in the intestine.

11. *Answer:* B
    Rationale: Clients with hematologic malignancies have oral problems, including stomatitis, two to three times more frequently than do clients with solid tumors.

12. *Answer:* C
    Rationale: This client needs aggressive oral care (q2–4h while awake). He may also have an infection. Lesions should be cultured, and appropriate medications (antibiotics, antifungals, antivirals) should be started. Steroids would further complicate the stomatitis rather than help.

13. *Answer:* B
    Rationale: Taste alterations can lead to anorexia, which can lead to negative nitrogen balance.

14. *Answer:* D
    Rationale: Spices and flavorings can enhance taste sensations altered by chemotherapy.

15. *Answer:* D
    Rationale: A decreased threshold for bitter tastes is related to negative nitrogen balance.

16. *Answer:* A
    Rationale: Commercial mouthwashes contain alcohol, which dries the mucosa and may lead to further taste changes as well as mucosal damage. Other interventions are useful in managing taste alterations.

17. *Answer:* C
    Rationale: Hypogeusia is the term for decreased taste sensation. Ageusia is absence of the taste sensation. Dysgeusia is an unusual (un-

pleasant) taste perception. Sialagogues are agents that affect salivary glands.

18. *Answer:* B
Rationale: Oral candidiasis occurs commonly and is associated with taste alterations. Gram-positive bacterial infections of the mouth occur infrequently. Herpes zoster, commonly known as shingles, does not generally involve the oral cavity; herpes simplex does.

19. *Answer:* B
Rationale: Psychogenic factors play a role in feelings of nausea. Anticipatory nausea or vomiting occurs in approximately 25% of chemotherapy clients.

20. *Answer:* A
Rationale: Medicating after vomiting does little to relieve the nausea that preceded the emesis.

21. *Answer:* D
Rationale: Areas that are quiet, cool, well-ventilated, and free of noxious sights and smells usually minimize nausea best.

22. *Answer:* A
Rationale: Persons most at risk for having chemotherapy-related nausea are younger clients, females, non-alcohol drinkers, non-drug users, and those with past history of motion sickness or emesis with pregnancy.

23. *Answer:* D
Rationale: There are many physiologic causes of nausea and vomiting, including all of the responses.

24. *Answer:* C
Rationale: Clients at risk for nausea should avoid lying down or reclining for at least 30 minutes after meals.

25. *Answer:* A
Rationale: Cisplatin has a high emetic potential (75%) related to stimulation of the chemoreceptor trigger zone (CTZ).

26. *Answer:* D
Rationale: All of these are potential sequelae of prolonged vomiting.

27. *Answer:* A
Rationale: Zofran commonly causes constipation, and stool softeners are often recommended, along with a high-fiber diet. Cisplatin generally causes nausea and vomiting for 24 to 120 hours, so Zofran is usually ordered for 24 to 48 hours around-the-clock after cisplatin administration. Sedation and extrapyramidal reactions are side effects of phenothiazine antiemetics but not of Zofran.

28. *Answer:* B
Rationale: Interferon and dacarbazine both can cause prolonged vomiting. There are many other pharmacologic and nonpharmacologic options for managing this client's symptoms. Allowing him to describe his symptoms may reveal clues as to which interventions might be most helpful. Anxiety and stress can affect these symptoms; however, they are not the only causes. Using one suppository after each emesis would not be effective and may result in overdose of Compazine.

29. *Answer:* C
Rationale: Classic steroid side effects are not seen when steroids are used short-term to manage nausea and vomiting.

30. *Answer:* D
Rationale: In palliative care, it is preferable to begin with a nonsedating phenothiazine or butyrophenone to manage symptoms, rather than inducing sedation. Other statements are correct.

31. *Answer:* C
Rationale: Lean body mass depletion, visceral mass depletion, and decreased functioning of the cellular and humoral immune systems can all be results of prolonged anorexia. Although bowel movements may be less frequent because of the lack of food intake, constipation is not a side effect of anorexia.

32. *Answer:* D
Rationale: Eating five servings of fruits and vegetables a day is healthy but will not prevent or diminish anorexia.

33. *Answer:* A
Rationale: Esophagitis is a side effect of chemotherapy or radiation, not dehydration.

34. *Answer:* B
Rationale: Multiple myeloma affects plasma cells and normally does not affect the neck or throat area.

35. *Answer:* D
Rationale: Sustacal is a caloric supplement, not a thickening agent.

36. *Answer:* B
Rationale: Mexican food is typically hot and spicy and may be difficult for a client to swallow.

37. *Answer:* C
Rationale: This is the correct definition.

38. *Answer:* A
Rationale: The other selections are associated with increased moisture. Although some of the foods a client may like may be moist, others may be dry, spicy, or hot and would irritate the oral mucosa.

39. *Answer:* C
Rationale: Stomatitis is mucositis of the oral cavity. Esophagitis is mucositis of the esophagus, and enteritis is mucositis of the intestines.

40. *Answer:* B
Rationale: Dysgeusia is defined as an unusual taste perception, perceived as unpleasant. Hypogeusia is a decrease in the acuity of the sensation of taste, and ageusia is an absence of the taste sensation.

41. *Answer:* C
Rationale: Although it would be unusual, changes in taste sensation can last for up to a year past therapy.

42. *Answer:* A
Rationale: This occurs with doses of more than 1 Gy of radiation and usually starts on day 10 to 14 and lasts for up to 21 days.

43. *Answer:* D
Rationale: Although clients may experience loss of appetite with paclitaxel, the other drugs—cisplatin, cyclophosphamide, and methotrexate—commonly affect taste.

44. *Answer:* B
Rationale: Infections in the mouth have been known to occur in up to 50% of neutropenic clients.

45. *Answer:* B
Rationale: Mucosal epithelial cells line the gastrointestinal tract, starting in the mouth and ending in the rectum.

46. *Answer:* B
Rationale: Soft or pureed foods are easier to swallow; liquids have an increased risk of being aspirated. The neck should never be hyperextended; it should be tilted forward if any position change is needed.

47. *Answer:* A
Rationale: Oral stomatitis can lead to swallowing difficulties.

48. *Answer:* B
Rationale: The role of a speech therapist includes assistance with swallowing problems.

49. *Answer:* C
Rationale: Potential complications of dysphagia include fluid and electrolyte imbalance, malnutrition, and aspiration.

50. *Answer:* D
Rationale: With tumor lysis syndrome, calcium is released from the intracellular compartment, producing hypercalcemia. Signs and symptoms include muscle cramps, flaccid paralysis, weakness, paresthesia, ECG changes, diarrhea, nausea, and bradycardia.

51. *Answer:* C
Rationale: Changes in mental status are some of the initial changes seen in clients with hypercalcemia.

52. *Answer:* C
Rationale: Signs and symptoms of hypokalemia include muscle weakness, a decrease in deep tendon reflexes, paresthesias, arrhythmias, mental confusion, lethargy, and apathy.

53. *Answer:* D
Rationale: Potassium-rich foods include bananas, oranges, potatoes, nuts, potato chips, fruit juices, broth, colas, and Gatorade.

54. *Answer:* C
   Rationale: At this level of hypercalcemia, symptoms would include muscle weakness and confusion. The nurse should encourage use of a bedside commode rather than a bedpan. In addition, transfer techniques to the bedside commode are safer than ambulation to the bathroom.

55. *Answer:* A
   Rationale: Metabolic alkalosis occurs when fluid volume is depleted and sodium, chloride, and potassium are lost.

56. *Answer:* C
   Rationale: Hypercalcemia of malignancy is frequently associated with high tumor burden and end-stage disease. Clients with lung and breast cancers account for the highest incidence rates. A common metastatic site of breast and lung cancers is bone.

57. *Answer:* A
   Rationale: Clients with breast cancer account for 20% to 40% of reported cases of hypercalcemia.

58. *Answer:* B
   Rationale: Hypercalcemia is the result of excessive bone resorption and impaired renal calcium excretion. Mobility and weight bearing are advocated.

59. *Answer:* B
   Rationale: Primary symptoms of SIADH are manifestations of water intoxication. Symptoms listed in responses A, C, and D are attributed to the effects of cerebral edema.

60. *Answer:* D
   Rationale: The key is signs of cachexia. The other answers may be symptoms of cachexia, but they are not warning signs.

61. *Answer:* C
   Rationale: Rapid infusion of enteral feedings overstimulates the gastrointestinal function, leading to the rapid excretion of the feeding through diarrhea.

BIBLIOGRAPHY

Berendt, M.C. (1998). Alterations in nutrition. In J. Itano & K. Taoka (eds.). *Core Curriculum for Oncology Nursing* (3rd ed.). Philadelphia: WB Saunders, pp. 223–258.

Foltz, A.T. (1997). Nutritional disturbances. In S. Groenwald, M. Frogge, M. Goodman, & C. Yarbro (eds.). *Cancer Nursing: Principles and Practice* (4th ed.). Boston: Jones & Bartlett, pp. 651–683.

Goodman, M., Hilderley, L.J., & Purl, S. (1997). Integumentary and mucous membrane alterations. In S. Groenwald, M. Frogge, M. Goodman, & C. Yarbro (eds.). *Cancer Nursing: Principles and Practice* (4th ed.). Boston: Jones & Bartlett, pp. 768–822.

14

Alterations in Elimination

April J. Dumond

Select the best answer for each of the following questions:

1. Mr. V. is a 68-year-old with prostate cancer. He has had a radical prostatectomy for stage III disease. He presents to the surgical oncology clinic for his 1-month follow-up and reports to the nurse that he has experienced urinary incontinence several times a day for the past week. Which statement, if made by Mr. V., indicates his understanding of his urinary symptoms?
   A. Urinary incontinence commonly occurs after removal of the prostate, so I will probably always be incontinent.
   B. The incontinence should have stopped by now, so I need to have an indwelling catheter, just like I did after my surgery.
   C. Urinary incontinence may continue for several months but should improve with a scheduled voiding program and pelvic muscle exercises.
   D. I need to take antibiotics, since my incontinence is probably caused by a bladder infection.

2. Mr. M., a 50-year-old with transitional cell carcinoma of the bladder, has received intravesical therapy with mitomycin. He is experiencing irritative bladder symptoms, including dysuria, daytime frequency, nocturia, and urgency. Which of the following is an appropriate outcome of symptom management for Mr. M.'s bladder disturbance?
   A. Voiding no more often than every hour during the day.
   B. Subjective report of relief from dysuria and bladder pain.

   C. Voiding no more than three times per night.
   D. Subjective report of urgent sensations less than three times per day.

3. Mrs. C. is a 61-year-old client with endometrial cancer. She recently underwent a total abdominal hysterectomy. She presents to the emergency department with a temperature of 101.2°F and complaints of severe dysuria, frequency, occasional urge incontinence, and low back pain. A urinalysis reveals the presence of WBCs and RBCs. Mrs. C. is prescribed trimethoprim-sulfamethoxazole (Bactrim DS) and phenazopyridine (Pyridium). Which of the following should *not* be included in the nurse's interactions with and teaching of the client?
   A. Verify that the client is not allergic to sulfa or other components of these medications.
   B. Inform her that her urine will turn orange-red and can stain her clothing.
   C. Limit oral fluids to 1500 mL/d or less.
   D. Do not use antacids concurrently; they decrease absorption of Bactrim.

4. Which of the following chemotherapy agents can cause neurotoxic side effects that may lead to difficulty or inability to reach the toilet before urination (functional incontinence)?
   A. Vincristine and vinblastine (Velban).
   B. 5-Fluorouracil (5-FU) and bleomycin.
   C. Methotrexate and doxorubicin (Adriamycin).
   D. Gemcitabine (Gemzar) and mitoxantrone (Novantrone).

5. Which of the following is a correct statement about the use of internal and external catheters to manage urinary incontinence?
   A. An internal or external catheter should be used at night to allow the client to get plenty of rest.
   B. Internal and external catheters should be used to prevent skin breakdown caused by incontinence.
   C. Catheters should never be used to manage incontinence.
   D. Catheters should be used as a last resort to manage incontinence.

6. Which of the following measures would be *most* appropriate to avoid perianal skin breakdown in the client with fecal incontinence?
   A. Always use a fecal incontinence pouch.
   B. Clean the perianal area after every voiding or bowel movement with a soft washcloth and perianal cleaner; rinse thoroughly and pat dry.
   C. Use warm sitz baths four times a day to prevent breakdown.
   D. Keep the client on a clear liquid diet to decrease frequency of stools.

7. Mrs. W. is a 53-year-old client with multiple myeloma who is currently harvesting peripheral stem cells for a future autologous transplantation. Today she reports pain in the lumbosacral spine, which she says was mild yesterday and now is severe, exacerbated by sitting up. She also states that she had urinary incontinence twice this morning and that she has not had a bowel movement for the past 3 days. Which is the *most* likely cause of Mrs. W.'s symptoms?
   A. Spinal cord compression as a complication of multiple myeloma.
   B. Immobility from lytic lesions, causing her to be unable to get to the toilet in time.
   C. Urinary tract infection.
   D. Metastatic brain lesions from multiple myeloma.

8. Ninety percent of all bowel obstructions occur in the
   A. sigmoid colon.
   B. transverse colon.
   C. small intestines.
   D. ascending colon.

9. Mr. D. is a 72-year-old with stage Dukes C colorectal cancer. He had a colon resection 2 years ago and has received 5-fluorouracil (5-FU) monthly since his surgery. He calls the cancer center and reports to the nurse that he has experienced constipation for the past few weeks. His last bowel movement was 4 days ago. He complains of abdominal distention, nausea, and onset of rectal bleeding this morning. Mr. D. is instructed to come to the clinic. What is the *most* likely cause of Mr. D's symptoms?
   A. Impaction from the constipating effects of 5-FU.
   B. Bowel obstruction, possibly from recurrent colorectal cancer.
   C. Change in dietary fiber intake and exercise.
   D. Chronic use of laxatives and enemas, which are no longer effective.

10. Mrs. H. is a 59-year-old client with advanced metastatic breast cancer. She is at home with hospice providing her care. She has severe bone pain and is taking opioids. Her daughter, who is her primary caregiver, states that Mrs. H. has begun to experience some constipation. Which statement indicates need for Mrs. H.'s daughter to have further instruction about a bowel program to prevent constipation?
    A. Mom needs to drink at least 8 glasses of fluid every day.
    B. Mom needs more fiber in her diet, like whole-grain cereals and breads, legumes, nuts, and fresh fruits and vegetables.
    C. Some light exercise such as walking may help to keep Mom regular.
    D. Magnesium citrate used daily will help to prevent constipation.

11. Ms O. is a 43-year-old client who has acute lymphocytic leukemia (ALL). She has completed induction therapy and is to begin consolidation with vincristine and prednisone. She has taken prednisone as part of earlier treatment. Information given to her about her new chemotherapy drug should include which of the following?
    A. Blood counts, especially the white blood cell count, may be affected.
    B. Peripheral neuropathies can occur.
    C. Bowel function should be monitored; stool softeners may be needed.
    D. All of the above.

12. Mr. J. has small cell lung cancer and is receiving combination chemotherapy. His blood counts today are WBC 800, platelets 32,000, hemoglobin 12.7, and hematocrit 38.1. He reports that he has not had a bowel movement for 3 days. Which of the following is an appropriate intervention for this client?
- A. Perform a rectal examination to check for impaction.
- B. Give Dulcolax 2 to 3 tabs orally, now and repeat this evening. If no relief is obtained within 24 hours, call the doctor.
- C. Administer soap-suds enemas until bowel is cleansed; then start stool softeners.
- D. Give glycerin suppositories to relieve constipation and continue daily to prevent recurrence of constipation.

13. Mrs. I. is a 39-year-old client with ovarian cancer. She has completed chemotherapy and has undergone a second-look operation, which revealed no evidence of malignancy. She presents to the clinic for the first postoperative visit with a complaint of constipation. Which of the following statements indicates that she needs further teaching?
- A. Surgery can cause constipation because of the handling of the intestines.
- B. My pain pills may cause me to be constipated. I should increase my fluid intake and take stool softeners.
- C. My cancer must have returned and caused my bowels to close off.
- D. I've not been very active since my surgery. Walking may help my bowels to move.

14. Which statement about use of laxatives is correct?
- A. All oral laxatives are contraindicated with suspected or actual intestinal obstruction because of the risk of bowel perforation.
- B. Lubricants coat and soften stool and can be used safely over the long term for bowel management.
- C. Enemas are effective for long-term bowel management.
- D. For clients with fluid restrictions, the best choice of laxative is a bulk-forming laxative such as Metamucil or Citrucel.

15. Mr. G. is a 63-year-old client with metastatic carcinoma of the colon. His disease is refractory to 5-FU. He received his first dose of irinotecan (Camptosar) 2 days ago. He began having diarrhea 36 hours after his therapy. Which of the following is an appropriate intervention for management of diarrhea in this client?
- A. Administer atropine to manage his diarrhea.
- B. Administer loperamide (Imodium-AD) and monitor closely for dehydration and fluid-electrolyte imbalances.
- C. Premedicate with dexamethasone before the next dose of irinotecan to prevent diarrhea.
- D. Diarrhea is an expected side effect and requires no management.

16. What is the *most common* side effect of opioid analgesics when used to manage cancer pain?
- A. Sedation.
- B. Slowed respiratory rate.
- C. Nausea and vomiting.
- D. Constipation.

17. Mrs. T. is a 45-year-old client with lymphoma who received an allogeneic bone marrow transplant 4 days ago. This morning she began to have large volumes of green, watery diarrhea. The BMT team visits her and explains that the diarrhea is caused by immunocompetent cells of the allogeneic donor marrow recognizing her normal gastrointestinal cells as "foreign." These cells initiate an immune reaction that attacks her gut. This condition is known as
- A. Crohn's disease.
- B. graft-versus-host disease.
- C. *Clostridium difficile.*
- D. Pseudomembranous colitis.

18. Which of these clients is at *greatest* risk for acute infectious diarrhea?
- A. Mr. K., a 36-year-old client who has HIV (human immunodeficiency virus) disease who just completed a 6-week course of antibiotics.
- B. Mrs. N., a 66-year-old client with acute myelogenous leukemia (AML), currently in remission, who is traveling in the northeastern United States.
- C. Miss B., an 8-year-old child, previously treated for rhabdomyosarcoma, in whom

there has been no evidence of disease for the past 3 years.

D. Mr. R., a 70-year-old client with prostate cancer, receiving intramuscular leuprolide (Lupron) monthly.

19. Mr. L., a 52-year-old client with rectal cancer, has completed the first 2 weeks of radiation therapy to the rectum. He began experiencing loose, watery stools 3 days ago. Which statement indicates that Mr. L. needs further instruction about managing his diarrhea?
   A. I should avoid foods high in fiber, fatty foods, and rich desserts.
   B. I will call the doctor if I have bloody or hard stools, can't keep down liquids, or have a temperature of 100.5°F or greater.
   C. I should drink less to make my bowel movements less watery.
   D. I can use Imodium-AD to control my diarrhea.

20. Which of the following biotherapy and chemotherapy agents is *most* likely to cause diarrhea?
   A. G-CSF (filgrastim, Neupogen).
   B. Carboplatin (Paraplatin).
   C. Dacarbazine (DTIC).
   D. Interferon.

21. The tumors that most commonly obstruct the bowel are
   A. hepatic and colorectal.
   B. ovarian and colorectal.
   C. ovarian and endometrial.
   D. pancreatic and ovarian.

22. Mrs. F. is a 43-year-old with advanced ovarian cancer. She presents to the clinic with complaints of abdominal distention, persistent cramping pain in the lower abdomen after eating, nausea, and no bowel movement for 3 days. On assessment, you note that the client has hypoactive bowel sounds. Which of the following does Mrs. F. most likely have?
   A. Partial bowel obstruction.
   B. Gastric outlet obstruction.
   C. Cholelithiasis.
   D. Bowel perforation with peritonitis.

23. Which factor is the *most* important in determining the consistency and volume of colostomy output?
   A. Amount and type of food eaten.
   B. Amount of fluid intake.
   C. Location of the colostomy on the abdomen.
   D. How much mucus is produced.

24. Which client undergoing surgery *most likely* would require a urinary diversion and a fecal diversion?
   A. 50-year-old man with abdominoperineal resection for colorectal cancer.
   B. 46-year-old woman with pelvic exenteration for extensive gynecologic cancer.
   C. 42-year-old man with low anterior colon resection for rectal cancer.
   D. 63-year-old woman with total abdominal hysterectomy with bilateral salpingo-oophorectomy.

25. Which type of cancer produces Bence Jones proteins and damaging casts that result in renal dysfunction, often requiring hemodialysis?
   A. Testicular cancer.
   B. Cervical cancer.
   C. Small cell lung cancer.
   D. Multiple myeloma.

26. Which of the following chemotherapy agents requires aggressive hydration before, during, and after therapy to prevent renal toxicity?
   A. Methotrexate.
   B. Cyclophosphamide (Cytoxan).
   C. Cisplatin.
   D. All of the above.

27. The following are potential complications of bowel obstruction *except*
   A. dehydration.
   B. peritonitis.
   C. fluid overload.
   D. bowel perforation.

28. Ms Q. has a new colostomy after a colon resection for a malignancy in the descending colon. She has just been discharged from the hospital. Which of these statements indicates that Ms Q. understands the care of her colostomy?
   A. I should change the appliance every day.
   B. I need to empty the pouch when it is about one third to one half full.

C. When I cut the pouch opening, the barrier should clear the stoma by about ½ inch, so the stoma is not rubbed by the appliance.
D. I will clean the stoma with peroxide to make sure all stool is removed.

29. Mrs. U. has breast cancer with bone metastases. Which condition commonly occurs with her disease and can cause the kidneys to lose the ability to concentrate urine?
   A. Hyperkalemia.
   B. Hypocalcemia.
   C. Hyponatremia.
   D. Hypercalcemia.

30. A critical change in the condition of a client with constipation that should be reported to the physician is
   A. inadequate fluid intake.
   B. absence of bowel sounds.
   C. cramping with enemas.
   D. failure to evacuate daily.

31. Which would be correct nutritional advice for a client prone to constipation?
   A. Keep foods soft and bland to avoid bowel irritation.
   B. Take all narcotics with milk to reduce the incidence of gastrointestinal upset.
   C. Maintain fluid intake of 1000 mL/d to prevent dehydration.
   D. Include foods high in fiber and roughage in daily diet.

32. Which medication could cause constipation?
   A. Chloral hydrate.
   B. Digoxin.
   C. Morphine.
   D. Daunorubicin.

33. Ms C. complains of abdominal bloating and cramping with no bowel movement for 5 days. She usually has a bowel movement every day. Bowel sounds are present. She received 80 mg of Adriamycin 10 days before this appointment. Recommendations include
   A. a soap-suds enema to relieve constipation immediately.
   B. a Fleets enema to stimulate peristalsis.
   C. an oral cathartic until bowel movement; then evaluate the need for daily stool softeners.

D. beginning daily stool softeners for constipation and mild narcotic for abdominal pain.

34. Mr. F. is receiving combination therapy of 5-fluorouracil and radiation for colorectal cancer. He is most at risk for which of the following side effects?
   A. Peripheral neuropathy.
   B. Alopecia.
   C. Thrombocytopenia.
   D. Diarrhea.

35. A nursing diagnosis related to diarrhea is alteration in protective mechanisms related to altered skin integrity. Which of the following nursing actions would correspond to this diagnosis?
   A. Applying zinc oxide ointment to the rectal area to protect skin.
   B. Applying a skin-barrier dressing to the rectal area to form a protective barrier.
   C. Avoiding sitz baths because they will promote bacterial growth.
   D. Cleansing the rectal area with water and mild soap after each bowel movement, rinsing well, and patting dry.

36. Diarrhea can lead to fluid and electrolyte imbalance. Which of the following imbalances is of particular concern?
   A. Hypokalemia.
   B. Hypercalcemia.
   C. Hypernatremia.
   D. Hyperkalemia.

37. Mrs. S. is receiving radiation therapy to her abdomen and asks for dietary instructions to decrease her diarrhea. You instruct her as follows.
   A. Eat a high-fiber diet that is high in protein.
   B. Eat what you want because diet has little or no effect on radiation-induced diarrhea.
   C. Begin a low-residue diet that is high in protein.
   D. Avoid solid foods and begin supplemental liquid feedings until diarrhea resolves.

38. Which of the following classes of chemotherapy drugs carries a high-risk potential for diarrhea?
   A. Vinca alkaloids.
   B. Antimetabolites.

C. Hormonal agents.

D. Nitrosoureas.

39. Ms L. is at the nadir of her chemotherapy regimen. She is occasionally incontinent of urine, and her family requests that a Foley catheter be inserted. You explain this would not be wise at this time because

A. Ms L. is at increased risk for infection.

B. it would be difficult for Ms L. to regain her bladder function.

C. Ms L. needs to become more independent with her daily activities.

D. the insertion of a Foley catheter would delay Ms L.'s discharge.

40. Mrs. S. is an elderly, alert woman with metastatic breast cancer. She was admitted to your unit for management of treatment-induced congestive heart failure. On admission she is given 80 mg of furosemide. Since she is elderly, frail, and in a strange environment, you are concerned about urinary incontinence. Your nursing plan would include

A. providing adult diapers for the client so she will not have to worry about incontinence.

B. inserting a Foley catheter to avoid incontinence.

C. placing a commode at the bedside and instructing the client in its use.

D. no special measures.

41. Mrs. P. is going home after a stay on the rehabilitation unit. She will be performing intermittent self-catheterization. Her discharge instructions include which of the following?

A. Use a new catheter with each catheterization.

B. Perform catheterization only when you feel the urge to void.

C. Expect scant amount of blood in the urine as normal and no cause for alarm.

D. Use catheters repeatedly as long as they are cleansed after each use.

42. Mrs. P. has urinary incontinence related to a central neurologic deficit. You are to begin a bladder training program with her in anticipa-

tion of discharge. Which of the following measures would be included in your program?

A. Maintain fluid intake at 1000 to 1500 mL/d.

B. Avoid measures that would artificially stimulate voiding.

C. Establish a voiding schedule, offering the bedpan every 2 hours.

D. Avoid intermittent catheterization to prevent infection.

43. When choosing an ostomy appliance for your client, which of the following should be considered?

A. Character of client's abdomen.

B. Location of stoma.

C. Character of stoma.

D. All of the above.

44. Mrs. J. has just undergone a cystectomy for bladder cancer and has an ileal conduit. As part of client teaching, the nurse should stress

A. changing the ostomy appliance just before bedtime.

B. attaching tubing every night for drainage.

C. removing the appliance for bathing.

D. using a permanent appliance that never needs changing.

45. The distal segment of the colon that is sutured to the abdominal wall in a double-barrel colostomy is also known as a

A. loop colostomy.

B. fascial bridge.

C. mucous fistula.

D. distal colostomy.

46. Which of the following is a risk factor that can lead to renal dysfunction?

A. Radiation therapy that may cause permanent fibrosis and atrophy.

B. Fluid and electrolyte imbalances from some chemotherapy drugs.

C. Compression by a metastatic tumor that may cause obstruction and hydronephrosis.

D. All of the above.

ANSWERS

1. *Answer:* C
   Rationale: Urinary incontinence is common after a radical prostatectomy. An indwelling catheter is usually left in place for a few weeks, and then bladder retraining is started. Some incontinence may persist for several months. Interventions may include establishing a schedule for voiding, gradually increasing the intervals between voiding, and pelvic muscle exercises.

2. *Answer:* B
   Rationale: Voiding should be no more often than every 2 hours during the day and no more than once per night for clients younger than 65 years of age. There should be no reports of dysuria, bladder pain, or urgent sensations.

3. *Answer:* C
   Rationale: Oral fluids should be increased to at least 2500 mL/d, rather than restricted, unless contraindicated (i.e., cardiac disease).

4. *Answer:* A
   Rationale: Vincristine and vinblastine can cause neurotoxic side effects that can lead to difficulty in reaching the toilet in time to urinate, also called functional incontinence.

5. *Answer:* D
   Rationale: Internal and external catheters are appropriate to manage incontinence in some circumstances but should be reserved as the last resort.

6. *Answer:* B
   Rationale: Good skin care after each voiding or stool will optimize the perianal skin integrity.

7. *Answer:* A
   Rationale: Multiple myeloma does not characteristically metastasize to the brain; rather myeloma can cause lesions in the spine, which can cause spinal cord compression. Spinal cord compression presents with back or neck pain as an early sign. Urinary incontinence and constipation are late signs, requiring immediate intervention.

8. *Answer:* C
   Rationale: Most obstructions occur in the small intestines, especially mechanical obstructions

such as adhesions, hernias, tumors, intussusception, inflammatory bowel disease, and strictures.

9. *Answer:* B
   Rationale: His symptoms are consistent with bowel obstruction, most likely recurrent colorectal cancer. Constipation is not a side effect of 5-FU therapy. Diarrhea is the more likely effect of 5-FU.

10. *Answer:* D
    Rationale: Magnesium citrate is of little to no use in prevention of constipation. Its primary use is in the acute evacuation of the bowel.

11. *Answer:* D
    Rationale: Vincristine side effects include neurotoxicity (peripheral neuropathies, cranial nerve neuropathy, CNS toxicity, constipation, paralytic ileus, and urinary retention), bone marrow suppression, extravasation, and hyperuricemia.

12. *Answer:* B
    Rationale: Rectal examinations, enemas, and suppositories are contraindicated in clients who are neutropenic or thrombocytopenic. An oral cathartic is indicated to give the client timely relief.

13. *Answer:* C
    Rationale: Constipation may be caused by manipulation of the intestines during surgery, use of analgesics and narcotics, and immobility. Obstruction of bowel by tumor can cause constipation, but it is not likely since her surgery showed no evidence of further disease.

14. *Answer:* A
    Rationale: Oral laxatives should never be used for actual or suspected intestinal obstruction. Lubricants, if used long term, can cause malabsorption of fat-soluble vitamins. Prolonged use of enemas can result in loss of normal bowel function and dependence. Bulk-forming laxatives are not an appropriate laxative choice for fluid-restricted clients, as they must be taken with a full glass of water.

15. *Answer:* B
    Rationale: Appropriate management of irinotecan-induced "late diarrhea" (occurring

more than 24 hours after treatment) is loperamide (Imodium-AD). Clients should be monitored closely for dehydration and fluid-electrolyte imbalances. Atropine, or Lomotil that contains atropine sulfate, is used to treat "early diarrhea" (occurring during first 24 hours after treatment). Dexamethasone as a premedication is used to prevent nausea and vomiting, not diarrhea.

16. *Answer:* D
Rationale: Constipation occurs in 40% of clients referred to a palliative care service and is the most common side effect from opioid therapy.

17. *Answer:* B
Rationale: Graft-versus-host disease occurs when the donor cells recognize the normal gastrointestinal cells as foreign. This condition can sometimes be prevented with immunosuppressive prophylaxis, such as cyclosporin A, corticosteroids, or other agents, or by T-cell depletion of donor marrow cells before infusion.

18. *Answer:* A
Rationale: The client with HIV disease is at greatest risk, since his immune system is incompetent. He also recently took antibiotics, which places him at risk for overgrowth of *Clostridium difficile* or other organisms. The AML and rhabdomyosarcoma survivors are in remission; therefore they are not at increased risk for infectious diarrhea. Ms N. is traveling in the northeastern United States. Although traveling can place individuals at increased risk for infectious diarrhea, it is less likely to occur than for travelers outside the United States. Lupron does not cause myelosuppression.

19. *Answer:* C
Rationale: The client should increase oral fluids, rather than restricting them, to avoid dehydration. A low-residue diet and Imodium-AD are used to manage radiation-induced acute diarrhea.

20. *Answer:* D
Rationale: Interferon commonly causes diarrhea. The other agents do not typically cause diarrhea. Carboplatin and DTIC are not biologic agents.

21. *Answer:* B
Rationale: Ovarian and colorectal cancers most commonly cause bowel obstruction.

22. *Answer:* A
Rationale: Her symptoms indicate a partial bowel obstruction. The characteristics of the client's pain are not consistent with bowel perforation and peritonitis, which cause a boardlike abdomen and increased pain on moving. Gastric outlet obstruction causes pain higher in the abdomen and sour emesis that is not bile-colored.

23. *Answer:* C
Rationale: The location of the colostomy is the main determining factor. A cecostomy or ascending colostomy produces semifluid or mushy stool. A transverse colostomy drains mushy stool. A descending or sigmoid colostomy produces soft to formed stool and can be regulated by irrigation.

24. *Answer:* B
Rationale: Pelvic exenteration involves removal of all reproductive organs and adjacent tissues and frequently requires both a colostomy and a urostomy because of advanced disease involvement of the colon, bladder, ureters, and other organs.

25. *Answer:* D
Rationale: Bence Jones proteins are found almost exclusively in the urine of clients with multiple myeloma. Renal insufficiency and renal failure are common with end-stage disease.

26. *Answer:* C
Rationale: Methotrexate's renal toxicity is dose related, and cyclophosphamide is more bladder toxic than renal toxic. Cisplatin requires aggressive hydration before, during, and after therapy.

27. *Answer:* C
Rationale: Fluid overload is not a possible complication of bowel obstruction.

28. *Answer:* B
Rationale: The pouch should be emptied before it is full. The appliance should be changed every 5 days or as needed because of leakage or skin discomfort, rather than every day. The pouch opening should be cut to allow $\frac{1}{8}$-inch clearance on sides of the stoma, rather than $\frac{1}{2}$ inch, which would expose too much skin. The stoma should be cleaned with water and patted dry, rather than cleaned with peroxide.

29. *Answer:* D
    Rationale: Hypercalcemia commonly occurs with metastatic breast cancer; multiple myeloma; squamous cell cancer of the lung, head, or neck; renal cell cancer; lymphomas; and leukemia. Hypercalcemia interferes with the kidneys' ability to concentrate urine.

30. *Answer:* B
    Rationale: Absence of bowel sounds may be a sign of obstruction, which is a potentially life-threatening complication.

31. *Answer:* D
    Rationale: Fluid intake should be 3000 mL, and diet should be high in fiber and roughage to stimulate peristalsis.

32. *Answer:* C
    Rationale: Narcotics can cause constipation.

33. *Answer:* C
    Rationale: Constipation of 3 days or more is unusual in this client and demands immediate relief. At 10 days after Adriamycin treatment, clients are susceptible to infection and should avoid rectal medications or treatments.

34. *Answer:* D
    Rationale: Combined 5-fluorouracil and abdominal radiation therapy have a synergistic effect to cause diarrhea.

35. *Answer:* D
    Rationale: The rectal area needs to be cleansed and dried to inhibit growth of bacteria. Sitz baths promote comfort.

36. *Answer:* A
    Rationale: Diarrhea results in potassium loss.

37. *Answer:* C
    Rationale: A low-residue diet will decrease irritation of the gastrointestinal tract.

38. *Answer:* B
    Rationale: Gastrointestinal alterations are a common toxicity of antimetabolites.

39. *Answer:* A
    Rationale: Indwelling Foley catheters are a source of infection.

40. *Answer:* C
    Rationale: The client should be near a commode for easy access and for measurement of urine output.

41. *Answer:* D
    Rationale: Self-intermittent catheterization is a clean, not sterile, technique.

42. *Answer:* C
    Rationale: A schedule is an integral part of a bladder-training program. The program also includes teaching measures to stimulate voiding and catheterizing client until residual is less than 50 mL after voiding.

43. *Answer:* D
    Rationale: The character of the client's abdomen and location and character of the stoma are important in determining the best type of ostomy appliance for the client.

44. *Answer:* B
    Rationale: For the bladder to drain continuously, the conduit must be drained at night. Attaching tubing to the appliance promotes drainage and prevents leakage.

45. *Answer:* C
    Rationale: The defunctionalized segment of colon is not removed and continues to produce mucus. The proximal bowel contains the functional stoma.

46. *Answer:* D
    Rationale: All of these risk factors can cause renal dysfunction.

BIBLIOGRAPHY

Agency for Health Care Policy and Research. (1996). *Managing Acute and Chronic Incontinence: Quick Reference Guide for Clinicians.* (AHCPR Publication No. 96-0686). Rockville, MD: United States Department of Health and Human Services.

Doughty, D., & Jackson, D. (1993). *Gastrointestinal Disorders.* St. Louis: Mosby–Year Book.

Hossan, E., & Striegel, A. (1993). Carcinoma of the bladder. *Semin Oncol Nurs 9*(4), 252–263.

Johnson, V., & Gary, A. (1995). Urinary incontinence: A review. *J Wound Ostomy Continence Nurs 1*(1), 8–15.

Kaplan, M. (1994). Hypercalcemia of malignancy: A review of advances in pathophysiology. *Oncol Nurs Forum 21*(6), 1039-1046.

Karlowicz, K. (1995). *Urologic Nursing Principles and Practice.* Philadelphia: WB Saunders.

McConnell, E.A. (1994). Loosening the grip of intestinal obstructions. *Nursing 24*(3), 32–42.

Marcio, J., Jorge, N., & Wexner, S. (1993). Etiology and management of fecal incontinence. *Dis Colon Rectum 36*(1), 77–97.

Ripamonti, C. (1994). Management of bowel obstruction in advanced cancer patients. *J Pain Symptom Manage 9*(3), 193–200.

Roberts, M.F. (1993). Diarrhea: A symptom. *Holist Nurs Pract 7*(2), 73–80.

Sangwan, Y., & Coller, J. (1994). Fecal incontinence. *Surg Clin North Am 74*(6), 1377–1398.

Walsh, B., Grunert, B., Teiford, G., & Otterson, M. (1995). Multidisciplinary management of altered body image in the patient with an ostomy. *J Wound Ostomy Continence Nurs 22*(9), 223–236.

Wright, P.S., & Thomas, S.L. (1995). Constipation and diarrhea: The neglected symptoms. *Semin Oncol Nurs 11*(4), 289–297.

NOTES

PART IV

Cardiopulmonary Function

15

Alterations in Ventilation

April J. Dumond

Select the best answer for each of the following questions:

1. Chemotherapy-induced pulmonary toxicity is a known side effect of which agent?
   A. 5-Fluorouracil (5-FU).
   B. Bleomycin (Blenoxane).
   C. Etoposide (VP-16).
   D. 6-Mercaptopurine (6-MP).

2. Which client would be at greatest risk for developing radiation-induced pneumonitis?
   A. 49-year-old man receiving radiation therapy for rectal cancer.
   B. 35-year-old woman with breast cancer, receiving radiation therapy after lumpectomy.
   C. 68-year-old man with recurrent lung cancer, previously treated with radiation therapy, currently receiving cisplatin and etoposide (VP-16).
   D. 52-year-old woman with multiple myeloma, receiving radiation therapy to treat spinal cord compression in the thoracic spine.

3. RBC transfusions are indicated for which client?
   A. Client with hemoglobin of 10 g/100 mL, experiencing dyspnea and tachycardia.
   B. Client with hemoglobin of 6.7 g/100 mL, without symptoms.
   C. Client with hemoglobin of 9.1 g/100 mL, experiencing epistaxis, hemoptysis, and melena.
   D. All of these clients.

4. Ms G. is a 43-year-old with recurrent breast cancer. She presents to the ambulatory cancer center with dyspnea and a dry, nonproductive cough. Her vital signs are temperature 100.4°F, pulse 88, respirations 42, and blood pressure of 110/76 mm Hg. On physical examination, Ms G. is noted to have diminished breath sounds and dullness to percussion on the right side, as well as a pleural friction rub. Her chest x-ray film shows blunting of the costophrenic angle. Ms G. is most likely experiencing which complication of her breast cancer?
   A. Malignant pleural effusion.
   B. Pneumothorax.
   C. Pneumonia.
   D. Superior vena cava syndrome.

5. Mr. B. is a 60-year-old with chronic myelogenous leukemia receiving oral hydroxyurea daily. The home health nurse monitors his CBC twice monthly. Last week, Mr. B.'s results were WBC 2.1, platelets 150,000, hemoglobin 8.6, hematocrit 25.8. His wife calls the home health agency, stating that Mr. B. is short of breath and confused this morning. He is afebrile and has no signs or symptoms of an infection. What problem is the client most likely experiencing?
   A. Thrombocytopenia with CNS bleeding.
   B. Anemia.
   C. Sepsis.
   D. Pneumonitis with pulmonary toxicity.

6. The most appropriate medical management intervention for the client receiving bleomycin

and at risk for chemotherapy-induced pulmonary toxicity is

A. discontinue the drug if dyspnea occurs and administer corticosteroids to control symptoms.
B. administer antibiotics to prevent pulmonary infections.
C. thoracentesis to remove effusion and attempt sclerotherapy to prevent further effusions.
D. prevent toxicity by monitoring baseline pulmonary function tests and limit cumulative dose of bleomycin to less than 400 units.

7. Client and family education regarding anemia should include

A. alternating activity and rest, and energy conservation.
B. safety precautions to prevent falls and injuries.
C. report change in mental status, increase in shortness of breath, and onset of active bleeding.
D. all of the above.

8. Mrs. W., a 53-year-old client with advanced endometrial cancer, is receiving methotrexate, dactinomycin, and cyclophosphamide (Cytoxan) every 21 days. She has experienced significant myelosuppression with previous courses of treatment, particularly anemia. Which biological response modifier may be ordered to prevent recurrence of anemia?

A. Recombinant human erythropoietin alfa (Procrit).
B. Granulocyte colony-stimulating factor (G-CSF or filgrastim/Neupogen).
C. Granulocyte macrophage colony-stimulating factor (GM-CSF or sargramostim/Leukine).
D. Recombinant human thrombopoietin (oprelvekin/Neumega).

9. Physical findings in the client experiencing dyspnea may include all of the following *except*

A. use of accessory muscles with breathing.
B. retraction of intercostal spaces.
C. slowed respiratory rate.
D. clubbing of digits caused by chronic hypoxemia.

10. Mrs. T. underwent a wedge resection for an isolated lesion of non-small cell lung cancer 6 weeks ago and is now neutropenic after receiving the second course of chemotherapy. Her temperature is 101.8°F, and a chest x-ray film indicates accumulation of fluid in the pleural space at the site of her resection. On thoracentesis, 60 mL of purulent fluid is noted. Mrs. T.'s condition is most likely

A. empyema.
B. hemothorax.
C. pneumothorax.
D. emphysema.

11. Ms J. had a central venous catheter placed this morning. Within an hour, she complained of shortness of breath and discomfort at the site of the catheter placement. The physician orders a STAT chest x-ray. Which condition should the nurse anticipate?

A. Pneumonia.
B. Superior vena cava syndrome.
C. Pleural effusion.
D. Pneumothorax.

12. Mr. S. has newly diagnosed non-small cell lung cancer, with lesions localized in the left upper and left lower lobes only. The surgical procedure that is most appropriate for Mr. S. is

A. wedge resection.
B. pneumonectomy.
C. lobectomy.
D. segmental resection.

13. Mrs. M. has non-small cell lung cancer and is receiving cyclophosphamide, doxorubicin, and cisplatin every 28 days. Her physician has ordered oxygen by nasal cannula at 1.5 L/min. When Mrs. M. arrives at the cancer center to receive her fourth course of therapy, you notice that her portable oxygen is set on 4 L/min. She tells you that her dyspnea has become more severe over the past few days and that she increased her oxygen flow rate. Your best response to Mrs. M. is

A. Since your shortness of breath has increased, it is okay to increase your oxygen until you can breathe better.
B. You should never increase your oxygen without asking the doctor first, since he may be angry that you didn't ask first.

C. Since your shortness of breath has increased, it is okay to increase your oxygen but not higher than 3 L/min.

D. Increasing your oxygen may be harmful to your lungs and your breathing. Tell me more about your shortness of breath.

14. To assess the extent of a client's dyspnea, which of the following questions would *not* be helpful?
   A. How many pillows do you use while sleeping?
   B. How many cigarettes do you smoke a day?
   C. Are you able to carry out your usual daily activities?
   D. Previously you could climb one flight of stairs comfortably. Can you still climb a flight of stairs?

15. Mr. V. previously received mitomycin for bladder cancer. His chemotherapy regimen was just changed to CMV (cisplatin, methotrexate, and vinblastine). When the vinblastine infusion begins, Mr. V. starts to experience acute shortness of breath and severe bronchospasm. The nurse's *first* intervention should be
   A. begin oxygen at 2 L/min.
   B. stop the vinblastine administration and assess for an open airway.
   C. call respiratory therapy to administer an updraft of a bronchodilator.
   D. administer decadron intravenously.

16. Early symptoms of radiation therapy–induced pulmonary toxicity may include all of the following *except*
   A. tachypnea and cyanosis.
   B. nonproductive cough.
   C. dyspnea.
   D. low-grade temperature.

17. The cardinal symptom of chemotherapy-induced pulmonary toxicity is
   A. malaise.
   B. fatigue.
   C. dyspnea.
   D. fever.

18. Education regarding energy conservation for clients with dyspnea should include all of the following *except*

A. alternate rest and activity, allowing frequent rest periods.
B. complete all activities of daily living in the morning before dyspnea and fatigue become worse.
C. simplify meal preparation and keep often-used items within reach.
D. use adaptive equipment for ADL, such as walkers, canes, reaching devices, and shower stools.

19. Agents that may be used for sclerotherapy, to prevent recurrent pleural effusions by producing mesothelial fibrosis, include all of the following *except*
   A. talc.
   B. tetracycline or doxycycline.
   C. bleomycin or nitrogen mustard.
   D. doxorubicin.

20. Closed chest drainage is not indicated after which type of chest surgery?
   A. Thoracotomy with wedge resection.
   B. Lobectomy.
   C. Pneumonectomy.
   D. Segmental resection.

21. Mr. C. is discharged to home after a thoracotomy with right upper lobectomy for lung cancer. Which statement indicates that the client needs more teaching about postoperative care?
   A. I should take deep breaths and cough regularly to loosen mucus.
   B. If it hurts when I cough, I should wait and cough later, when the pain lessens.
   C. If I have pain when I deep breathe and cough, I should take my pain medicine, so I can continue to do my breathing exercises.
   D. If I cough up yellow or brown mucus, I should call the doctor.

22. Which diagnostic test would be most helpful to identify early signs of pulmonary toxicity caused by chemotherapeutic agents such as bleomycin and carmustine (BCNU)?
   A. Pulmonary function tests (PFTs).
   B. Ventilation-perfusion scan.
   C. Arterial blood gases (ABGs).
   D. Chest x-ray examination.

23. Mrs. E. is a 62-year-old client with breast cancer, metastatic to the lungs. She reports that she has a lot of dyspnea at night. Which statement best indicates Mrs. E.'s understanding of her care in managing dyspnea?
    A. I should keep the head of the bed down, to make breathing easier.
    B. I will take twice my usual dose of pain medicine at bedtime, so I will have less shortness of breath.
    C. I can elevate the head of the bed or use extra pillows to help me breathe easier.
    D. I should increase my oxygen to a higher flow rate at bedtime.

24. Which of the following is least likely to cause hypoventilation?
    A. Primary or metastatic cancer of the lung.
    B. Immobility.
    C. Tumor debulking surgery for head and neck cancer.
    D. History of diabetes.

25. Ms F. has a tracheostomy. She reports that her secretions are thick and that she has difficulty coughing productively. Which statement indicates that Ms F. needs more teaching?
    A. I should use humidified air or oxygen by tracheostomy collar to keep the mucosa and secretions from drying.
    B. I will drink at least 8 glasses of liquids every day.
    C. I must get a flu shot and a pneumococcal vaccine each year to help prevent flu and pneumonia.
    D. I should avoid crowds during flu and cold season.

26. Abnormal accumulation of blood within the pleural space is
    A. pneumothorax.
    B. hemothorax.
    C. hemoptysis.
    D. empyema.

27. Mr. O., who has newly diagnosed non-Hodgkin's lymphoma, is receiving his first course of ABVD therapy (doxorubicin, bleomycin, vinblastine, and dacarbazine). During therapy he has shortness of breath, wheezing, urticaria, and chills. Interventions to treat Mr. O.'s hypersensi-

tivity reaction should be implemented in which order of priority?
    A. Stop drug, assess airway, then give epinephrine and oxygen.
    B. Assess airway, give oxygen, stop drug, then give epinephrine.
    C. Give epinephrine, stop drug, assess airway, then give oxygen.
    D. Give oxygen, assess airway, give epinephrine, stop drug.

28. Mrs. R. has advanced breast cancer with lung metastasis. She tells you that she is having increasing shortness of breath, and she is afraid of dying. She asks, "Am I just going to smother to death?" The nurse's best response is
    A. I'll tell your doctor that you want to discuss your breathing problem.
    B. Tell me more about your shortness of breath and how it makes you feel.
    C. Yes, your breathing will become more and more labored, and you eventually will be unable to breathe at all.
    D. Would you like to see your pastor or the hospital chaplain?

29. Ms N., a 41-year-old with metastatic ovarian cancer, reports she has a history of panic attacks. She smokes 2 packs of cigarettes per day and has smoked for 20 years. Her lung metastasis has become symptomatic recently, and she tells the nurse that she seems to always have a panic attack when she is short of breath. Your instruction should include
    A. use oxygen whenever dyspnea occurs but do not turn the liter flow higher than 5 L/min.
    B. take Valium or Xanax whenever a panic attack occurs.
    C. stop smoking "cold turkey" to prevent further lung damage.
    D. use techniques for relaxation and controlled breathing, such as pursed-lip breathing and prolonged exhalation.

30. You are working the evening shift on the oncology unit. You are assigned eight clients, including Mr. H., a 62-year-old man with acute leukemia, receiving day 23 of DVPA induction chemotherapy (asparaginase, daunorubicin, prednisone, and vincristine); Mrs. J., a 53-year-old client with recurrent pleural effusions from metastatic breast cancer, who had sclerotherapy

with tetracycline this morning; Ms F., a 31-year-old client with newly diagnosed ovarian cancer, receiving her first course of paclitaxel (Taxol), which was begun 30 minutes ago; and Mr. M., a 25-year-old client with testicular cancer receiving his fourth course of BEP (bleomycin, etoposide, and cisplatin). Which of these clients is at highest risk for respiratory compromise and should be assessed first?

A. Mr. H.
B. Mrs. J.
C. Ms F.
D. Mr. M.

31. Which of the following positions would be most beneficial in decreasing the work of breathing?

A. Sitting in a chair with shoulders erect and pushed backward.
B. Sitting in a chair with shoulders relaxed and rolled forward.
C. Sitting in bed with the head of the bed elevated 25 degrees.
D. Sitting in bed with the head of the bed elevated 75 degrees.

32. Which of the following breathing techniques is most likely to improve the efficiency of the client's breathing?

A. Exhaling through the nose.
B. Exhaling through pursed lips.
C. Exhaling one half as long as inhaling.
D. Exhaling using accessory muscles.

33. Which of the following assessments would be most accurate in evaluating the severity of a client's dyspnea?

A. Respiratory rate and depth.
B. Use of accessory muscles for breathing.
C. Ability of the client to accomplish activities of daily living.
D. The client's perception of the amount of difficulty in breathing.

34. In preparing Mrs. C., a client experiencing dyspnea, for discharge from the hospital, the nurse evaluates the effectiveness of client and family teaching. Which of the following statements, if made by Mrs. C., would indicate a need for additional teaching?

A. If I have trouble breathing, I will just lie down with my head elevated on several pillows.

B. I will keep the temperature in the house a few degrees higher than usual.
C. I will arrange for a friend to be available if I need someone.
D. If I notice a big change in my dyspnea, I will call my doctor.

35. Which of the following dietary recommendations should the nurse make to increase the intake of nutrients needed for erythropoiesis?

A. Milk, eggs, liver, and green leafy vegetables.
B. Apples, peanuts, oats, and cottage cheese.
C. Cantaloupe, lima beans, and sweet potatoes.
D. Dry yeast, grapefruit, and tuna fish.

36. Mrs. M. has completed a 6-week course of radiation therapy to the mediastinum. She currently has a hemoglobin of 7.5. In evaluating the effectiveness of discharge teaching, which of the following comments, if made by Mrs. M., would indicate a need for additional instruction?

A. I should eat foods high in protein, iron, and vitamin B_{12}.
B. If I notice any dizziness, I should avoid driving the car.
C. I may not be able to do all my housework and go to work, too.
D. If I notice any palpitations, I will just lie down for awhile.

37. Mrs. J. has a hemoglobin of 6.5. She is experiencing symptoms of cerebral tissue hypoxia. Which of the following nursing interventions would be most important in providing care for Mrs. J.?

A. Providing rest periods throughout the day.
B. Instituting energy conservation techniques.
C. Assisting in ambulation to bathroom.
D. Checking temperature of water before bathing.

38. Mrs. C. is receiving radiation therapy to the pelvis for cancer of the cervix. Her hemoglobin is 7.0. Which of the following symptoms expressed by Mrs. C. would be indicative of tissue hypoxia related to anemia?

A. Dizziness.
B. Fatigue relieved by rest.
C. Skin that is warm to the touch.
D. Apathy.

ANSWERS

1. *Answer:* B
Rationale: Pulmonary toxicity occurs in approximately 10% of clients treated with bleomycin, beginning with pneumonitis and progressing to pulmonary fibrosis. It is dose related and occurs most frequently in clients who have received a cumulative dose in excess of 400 units.

2. *Answer:* C
Rationale: Risk factors for radiation-induced pneumonitis are concurrent chemotherapy, previous radiation therapy, and steroid withdrawal, and it tends to be more severe in the elderly.

3. *Answer:* D
Rationale: RBC transfusions are indicated for symptomatic anemia, regardless of the hemoglobin or hematocrit; active bleeding; and hemoglobin less than 8 g/100 mL.

4. *Answer:* A
Rationale: Malignant pleural effusions are often accompanied by fever, tachypnea, dyspnea, nonproductive cough, diminished or absent breath sounds, dullness to percussion, and pleural friction rub. Other findings may include chest pain, restricted chest wall expansion, and egophony on the affected side and may include mediastinal shift if the pleural effusion is severe.

5. *Answer:* B
Rationale: Mr. B.'s recent blood counts indicate that his hemoglobin and hematocrit may have fallen. The most likely cause of his symptoms is chemotherapy-related anemia, which frequently presents with changes in mental status and increased shortness of breath.

6. *Answer:* D
Rationale: The best treatment of pulmonary toxicity is prevention by monitoring baseline pulmonary function tests (PFTs) and limiting the cumulative bleomycin dose to less than 400 units. The proper treatment of bleomycin-induced pulmonary toxicity is correctly listed in response A (discontinue bleomycin, begin corticosteroids). Pneumonitis and fibrosis, rather than effusions, are typically seen with this toxicity.

7. *Answer:* D
Rationale: All of these should be included in client teaching about anemia.

8. *Answer:* A
Rationale: Recombinant erythropoietin (Procrit, also called EPO or Epogen) is indicated for the treatment of anemia related to myelosuppressive chemotherapy. G-CSF and GM-CSF are indicated for prevention of infection, and Neumega is indicated for the prevention and treatment of thrombocytopenia.

9. *Answer:* C
Rationale: Findings associated with dyspnea include all except slowed respiratory rate. Instead, tachypnea occurs, as well as increased respiratory excursion, flaring of nostrils, cyanosis, and pallor.

10. *Answer:* A
Rationale: Empyema is defined as the abnormal accumulation of infected fluid or pus in the pleural space as a result of recent chest surgery, immunocompromise, or lung infections.

11. *Answer:* D
Rationale: Symptoms are related to pneumothorax from central venous catheter placement. Dyspnea generally occurs as the pneumothorax increases in size.

12. *Answer:* B
Rationale: A pneumonectomy, the surgical removal of an entire lung, is indicated for this client. The term lobectomy refers to the removal of a single lobe. Wedge and segmental resections are removal of portions of a lobe.

13. *Answer:* D
Rationale: Higher flow rates of oxygen can be harmful for clients, especially those with chronic obstructive pulmonary disease (COPD), as it may decrease the central nervous system response to hypoxia (i.e., client's "drive" to breathe). The nurse should further assess the client's symptoms and discuss them with the physician.

14. *Answer:* B
Rationale: Good measures of dyspnea in-

clude the number of pillows used for sleeping or comfort and ability to carry out activities of daily living. Also, comparing the ability to do physical activity with previous levels of activity is helpful. Smoking habits may influence respiratory effort, but it is not generally directly related to amount of dyspnea.

15. *Answer:* B
Rationale: Although all of these interventions may be used to alleviate the client's symptoms, the nurse's first response should be to discontinue the administration of vinblastine and assess for an open airway. This hypersensitivity reaction can occur in clients receiving a vinca alkaloid who previously were treated with mitomycin (or are receiving concurrent therapy with mitomycin). Onset may be within minutes to hours after the vinca alkaloid.

16. *Answer:* A
Rationale: Tachypnea and cyanosis are late symptoms associated with radiation therapy–induced pulmonary toxicity.

17. *Answer:* C
Rationale: All of these symptoms occur; however, dyspnea is the cardinal symptom.

18. *Answer:* B
Rationale: Alternating rest with activity is essential to prevent severe dyspnea. Trying to complete all ADL at once may worsen symptoms.

19. *Answer:* D
Rationale: Doxorubicin (Adriamycin) is not used as a sclerosing agent because of its vesicant properties.

20. *Answer:* C
Rationale: Chest tubes are used to remove excess fluid and allow the remaining lung to reexpand and maximize lung function. With a pneumonectomy, an entire lung is removed. Therefore it is not necessary to use chest tubes. The fluid and blood consolidate and fill the space previously occupied by the removed lung tissue.

21. *Answer:* B
Rationale: Clients should be instructed to take pain medication when they hurt to enable them to continue to take deep breaths, cough, and be active. If they withhold analgesics, they

take shallow breaths, allowing secretions to pool and placing the clients at risk for atelectasis and infection.

22. *Answer:* A
Rationale: The earliest sign of pulmonary toxicity is dyspnea. Although dyspnea is a subjective symptom, pulmonary function tests can best detect early and subtle changes in respiratory function that other diagnostic tests may not show.

23. *Answer:* C
Rationale: Extra pillows and elevation of the head of the bed may provide comfort and ease dyspnea. Double doses of pain medication may depress respirations. High oxygen flow rates can suppress the respiratory drive.

24. *Answer:* D
Rationale: Risk factors for hypoventilation include primary or metastatic lung cancer, recent surgery, immobility, thoracic or head and neck surgery, surgery for palliation or tumor debulking, history of obstructive or restrictive pulmonary disease, and history of cardiovascular disease.

25. *Answer:* C
Rationale: Clients at higher risk for respiratory infections should consider getting the influenza vaccine each year; however, one pneumococcal vaccine protects clients for a lifetime. Revaccination may induce severe reactions because of high antibody titers, and there is evidence that booster vaccinations do not elevate antibody titers.

26. *Answer:* B
Rationale: Hemothorax is accumulation of blood in the pleural space.

27. *Answer:* A
Rationale: The drug should be stopped immediately to prevent further reaction. Simultaneously the nurse should assess for a patent airway. Then the nurse should administer epinephrine, oxygen, vasopressors, and intravenous fluid, as ordered.

28. *Answer:* B
Rationale: Although referring the client to a chaplain or to the physician may be helpful, Mrs. R. has verbalized her fears to the nurse. Allowing the client to ventilate her concerns and fears is the most therapeutic intervention.

29. *Answer:* D

Rationale: Breathing techniques and relaxation would be most beneficial for this client. Anxiolytics also may be helpful; however, taking them whenever a panic attack occurs may result in overdosage and should not be the first treatment option. Oxygen flow rate is too high for a smoker with preexisting lung disease. Smoking cessation is a priority, but quitting "cold turkey" may produce more anxiety; teaching should include possible options for smoking cessation, considering the client's history of panic attacks.

30. *Answer:* C

Rationale: Ms F. is at greatest risk and should be assessed first. She is receiving her first course of Taxol, which can cause hypersensitivity/anaphylaxis, with symptoms (dyspnea, chest pain, rash, and others) usually occurring within the first hour of the infusion. Mr. H., receiving day 23 of DVPA, has already received 6 days of asparaginase, which can cause anaphylaxis with bronchospasms; however, if he has not had symptoms of allergic reactions with prior doses, he will not likely have anaphylaxis with this dose. Mrs. J. had sclerotherapy several hours ago, so she mostly likely is not in acute distress; however, she should be assessed soon. Mr. M. is receiving his fourth round of bleomycin; allergic reactions or anaphylaxis generally occurs during the first or second dose, so he should be stable.

31. *Answer:* B

Rationale: The work of breathing is reduced by decreasing the resistance against which the respiratory muscles must work.

32. *Answer:* B

Rationale: Dyspnea is a distressing and powerless experience for clients. Concrete nursing interventions to modify the experience of, and the reaction to, dyspnea are important. With pursed-lip breathing, back pressure is created to keep airways open. This promotes more complete exhalation and facilitates removal of secretions from the tracheobronchial tree.

33. *Answer:* D

Rationale: Dyspnea is a subjective complaint. Other parameters may be indexes of the compromise of oxygenation and endurance, but client perception of severity is the most accurate index of severity.

34. *Answer:* B

Rationale: Breathing is easier in a cooler environment.

35. *Answer:* A

Rationale: Foods high in protein, vitamins, B_{12}, folic acid, and iron are needed for erythropoiesis.

36. *Answer:* D

Rationale: Palpitation is a significant change in the condition of the client and may be indicative of progressing anemia. Therefore, the client should report the symptom to the physician.

37. *Answer:* C

Rationale: Cerebral tissue hypoxia is commonly associated with dizziness. The greatest risk to the client with dizziness is potential injury, especially with changes in position.

38. *Answer:* A

Rationale: Cerebral tissue hypoxia is commonly associated with dizziness. Recognition of cerebral hypoxia is critical since the body will attempt to shunt oxygenated blood to vital organs.

BIBLIOGRAPHY

Davey, S.S., & McCance, K.L. (1994). Alterations of pulmonary function. In K.L. McCance & S.E. Huether (eds.). *Pathophysiology: The Biologic Basis for Disease in Adults and Children* (2nd ed.). St. Louis: Mosby–Year Book.

Ewald, G.S., & McKenzie, C.R. (eds.). (1995). *Manual of Medical Therapeutics* (28th ed.). Boston: Little, Brown.

Gross, J., & Johnson, B.L. (1993). *Handbook of Oncology Nursing* (2nd ed.). Sudbury, MA: Jones & Bartlett.

Groenwald, S.L., Frogge, M.H., Goodman, M., & Yarbro, C.H. (1993). *Cancer Nursing Principles and Practice* (3rd ed.). Sudbury, MA: Jones & Bartlett.

Pina, E.M., Harvey, J.C., Katariya, K., & Beattie, E.J. (1993). Malignant pleural effusions. In J.C. Harvey & E.J. Beattie (eds.). *Cancer Surgery.* Philadelphia: WB Saunders.

Stover, D.E. (1993). Pulmonary toxicity. In V.T. DeVita Jr., S. Hellman, & S.A. Rosenberg (eds.). *Cancer: Principles and Practice of Oncology* (4th ed.). Philadelphia: JB Lippincott, pp. 2362–2370.

16

Alterations in Circulation

Mary Mrozek-Orlowski

Select the best answer for each of the following questions:

1. Lymphedema is defined as
   A. bilateral swelling in the lower extremities.
   B. unilateral difference in affected limb of greater than 1.5 cm when compared with unaffected limb.
   C. unilateral swelling of an extremity that must have alteration in skin integrity.
   D. erythema in an affected extremity

2. Lymphedema can be worsened by which of the following?
   A. Radiation therapy to or infection in the affected extremity.
   B. Administration of chemotherapy in the unaffected arm.
   C. Application of an elastic sleeve to affected extremity.
   D. Administration of oral antibiotics.

3. Cancers that are associated with lymphedema include
   A. breast and prostate cancer.
   B. leukemia.
   C. any cancer in which axillary or groin lymph fluid flow is impaired by surgical scarring or metastatic tumor.
   D. basal cell skin carcinoma.

4. When assessing clients at risk for lymphedema, inspection of the affected extremity includes all of the following *except*
   A. condition of the skin.
   B. loss of hair on the extremity.

   C. impairment of circulation or constriction by clothing or jewelry.
   D. mobility of the extremity.

5. Severe lymphedema is classified as
   A. circumferential measurement of the affected extremity that is 5 cm greater than the unaffected extremity.
   B. tight, shiny skin with bilateral lower extremity edema.
   C. unilateral erythema and edema on the affected extremity.
   D. measurement of the affected extremity is 3 to 5 cm greater than the unaffected extremity.

6. Interventions and education aimed at preventing lymphedema in affected extremities include all of the following *except*
   A. prompt treatment of cuts and suspected infection.
   B. teaching clients to avoid lifting heavy objects such as suitcases with the affected arm.
   C. routine exercises to maintain range of motion.
   D. prophylactic antibiotics to prevent infection.

7. Early detection and treatment of lymphedema involves
   A. regular measurement of extremities and application of elastic sleeves when lymphedema occurs.
   B. massage therapy and vigorous weight lifting in the affected extremity.

C. weight lifting in the affected extremity and antibiotics.

D. referral to rehabilitation.

8. Treatment of chronic lymphedema includes interventions used in treatment of early lymphedema and

    A. application of fentanyl patch for pain control.

    B. avoiding use of narcotics because of fear of addiction.

    C. interventions to counter the negative effect of chronic lymphedema on activities of daily living and general functioning.

    D. vigorous exercise in the affected extremity.

9. Cardiovascular toxicity in clients receiving treatment for cancer is defined as

    A. alteration in cardiac conduction and function that is related to cancer treatment.

    B. increased risk of myocardial infarction related to years of untreated hypertension.

    C. unilateral lower extremity edema related to deep vein thrombosis.

    D. asymptomatic bradycardia.

10. High-dose cyclophosphamide is associated with which cardiac toxicity?

    A. Asymptomatic bradycardia.

    B. Coronary artery spasm.

    C. Cardiomyopathy.

    D. Endothelial damage leading to myocardial necrosis.

11. Asymptomatic bradycardia is related to which of the following chemotherapy agents?

    A. Daunorubicin.

    B. Methotrexate.

    C. Paclitaxel.

    D. None of the above.

12. Cardiac toxicities that begin several weeks after chemotherapy administration are most likely

    A. chronic.

    B. subacute.

    C. acute.

    D. not reversible.

13. The most common and well-known chronic cardiac toxicity is

    A. cardiomyopathy.

    B. asymptomatic bradycardia.

    C. hemorrhagic myocardial necrosis.

    D. coronary artery spasm.

14. Factors that are associated with increased risk of cardiotoxicity from cancer chemotherapy include

    A. high-dose cyclophosphamide, radiation therapy to the left thorax, and multiple cardiotoxic drugs.

    B. standard dose cyclophosphamide, being elderly, and history of smoking.

    C. history of smoking, bone metastases, and clients with lung cancer.

    D. high-dose cyclophosphamide, radiation therapy to left thorax, and history of breast cancer.

15. Tissue sensitivity and regimen intensity are cardiac risk factors in

    A. clients with melanoma.

    B. pediatric clients with cancer.

    C. the elderly.

    D. women with breast cancer treated with autologous bone marrow transplantation.

16. The administrative schedules of chemotherapy that increase risk of cardiotoxicity include

    A. high doses of drug over short periods of time.

    B. low doses of drug administered rapidly.

    C. 24-hour administration for head and neck cancer.

    D. combination administration of chemotherapy.

17. Nursing actions associated with the administration of cardiotoxic chemotherapy include all of the following *except*

    A. cardiac assessment of rate, rhythm, and regularity.

    B. notation in client chart of cumulative dose of anthracycline.

    C. assessment that ejection fraction and electrocardiogram results are within normal limits at the initiation of therapy.

    D. chest radiograph before surgery.

18. Laboratory values that can interfere with cardiac function when they are abnormal include

    A. sodium and calcium.

    B. potassium and chloride.

    C. potassium and calcium.

    D. sodium and chloride.

19. Tachycardia, shortness of breath, and neck vein distention are cardiac signs and symptoms of which of the following?
   A. Lung cancer.
   B. Congestive heart failure.
   C. Cardiomegaly.
   D. Impending cardiac arrest.

20. An appropriate nursing outcome for clients with cardiac toxicity related to cancer treatments is
   A. client will maintain activity levels that allow normal daily activities as identified by the client.
   B. client will experience no pain.
   C. client and caregiver will express relief at cancer cure.
   D. client will experience no dyspnea.

21. Dexrazoxane is an iron-chelating agent that is
   A. a cardioprotective agent used in pediatric clients.
   B. a kidney-protective agent indicated for use in clients receiving cisplatin.
   C. a cardioprotective agent used in breast cancer clients with metastatic disease who have received greater than 300 mg/m² of doxorubicin.
   D. an antiemetic agent used in regimens with high emetic potential.

22. Prevention of doxorubicin-related CHF cardiotoxicity includes
   A. exercise and smoking.
   B. cessation of smoking and oxygen therapy.
   C. exercise and administration of dexrazoxane as indicated.
   D. oxygen therapy and low-fat diet.

23. Talking with clients and families about energy conservation strategies is an example of
   A. client education for those at risk for, or who are experiencing congestive heart failure.
   B. prevention of cardiotoxicity.
   C. client education about signs of cardiotoxicity.
   D. community education.

24. When the ejection fraction is less than 50% to 55% of institutional normal values, health care providers should consider
   A. increasing the chemotherapy dose because it is not effective in eliminating cancer cells.

   B. reducing the chemotherapy dose because the client is at risk for cardiotoxicity.
   C. monitoring electrocardiograms.
   D. adding fluid to chemotherapy treatments because client is dehydrated.

25. Abnormal leakage of fluid from blood and lymph vessels leading to an excessive accumulation of fluid in interstitial spaces is defined as
   A. lymphedema.
   B. edema.
   C. hematoma.
   D. hepatoma.

26. Lymphatic capillaries function to
   A. remove excess fluid and protein from bloodstream.
   B. act as primary vessels returning blood to the heart.
   C. normalize balance of fluid between interstitial and intravascular spaces.
   D. promote fluid return from lower extremities.

27. Edema results from all of the following *except*
   A. interruption of lymph flow.
   B. vascular obstruction.
   C. any factor interfering with the balance of fluid flow between intravascular and interstitial spaces.
   D. excess water intake.

28. Decreased protein intake (i.e., malnutrition) and loss of serum protein (i.e., anemia and bleeding) are causes of
   A. decreased capillary fluid pressure.
   B. increased peripheral fluid pressure.
   C. obstructed lymphatics drainage.
   D. decreased capillary oncotic pressure.

29. Venous obstruction resulting in edema is caused by which of the following?
   A. Malignant tumor or thrombophlebitis.
   B. Cellulitis.
   C. Nausea and vomiting.
   D. Chemotherapy.

30. Increased dietary sodium and inadequate dietary protein are examples of which type of risk factor for malignant edema?
   A. Treatment.
   B. Iatrogenic.

C. Lifestyle.

D. Disease.

31. Objective findings related to malignant edema include
    A. 10-pound weight gain and pitting edema in lower extremities.
    B. bilateral edema of the extremities.
    C. diminished peripheral pulses in involved extremity.
    D. all of the above.

32. Which of the following statements regarding malignant pericardial effusions is true?
    A. Most are symptomatic.
    B. Testicular cancer is a common cause of pericardial effusion.
    C. Pericardial effusion is classified as an oncologic emergency.
    D. Pericardial effusions are always associated with pleural effusions.

33. Peritoneal effusions are caused by
    A. tumor seeding the peritoneum, leading to obstruction of lymphatics and increased capillary leakage of proteins and fluids into the peritoneum.

B. lymphoma.

C. a history of pleural effusions.

D. receiving a lifetime dose of doxorubicin.

34. Symptoms and findings suggestive of peritoneal effusion include
    A. infrequent urination.
    B. diarrhea.
    C. shortness of breath.
    D. chest pain.

35. Thrombotic events are associated with
    A. fluid collection in the lower extremities.
    B. paraneoplastic syndromes, metastatic cancer, and cancer treatments.
    C. ascites.
    D. mitomycin C.

36. Laboratory findings of thrombotic events are
    A. bruising.
    B. severe anemia and thrombocytosis (platelet count >400,000/µl).
    C. normal venograms of the affected extremities.
    D. visible blood in the stool.

NOTES

ANSWERS

1. *Answer:* B
   Rationale: Bilateral swelling in the lower extremities is defined as edema. Alteration in skin integrity is possible with lymphedema but is not necessarily present. Erythema in an affected extremity is suggestive of infection.

2. *Answer:* A
   Rationale: Radiation therapy worsens lymphedema by causing fibrosis and scarring in an extremity where lymph flow is already impaired by surgery. Infection worsens lymphedema by causing swelling associated with inflammation. All other answers are actions that either treat or prevent lymphedema.

3. *Answer:* C
   Rationale: Although breast and prostate cancer are associated with lymphedema, lymphedema can occur with any cancer or related sequela that obstructs lymph flow.

4. *Answer:* B
   Rationale: Although loss of hair is part of inspection, it is not a common finding in lymphedema.

5. *Answer:* A
   Rationale: Tight, shiny skin and bilateral edema are seen in cardiac disease and malignant pedal edema.

6. *Answer:* D
   Rationale: Lymphedema may be related to subclinical lymphangitis, and prompt treatment may prevent long-term sequelae. Maintaining an exercise routine strengthens muscles that facilitate lymph flow from the extremities.

7. *Answer:* A
   Rationale: Regular measurements of the extremities allow early detection of lymphedema and early application of elastic sleeves. Massage therapy is also helpful, but lifting heavy weights can worsen lymphedema.

8. *Answer:* C
   Rationale: Narcotics may be necessary for discomfort related to lymphedema; they should never be withheld for fear of addiction. Range of motion and gentle strength building may help, but vigorous exercise may worsen lymphedema.

9. *Answer:* A
   Rationale: Cancer therapies affect cardiac function and conduction.

10. *Answer:* D
    Rationale: High-dose cyclophosphamide used in bone marrow and stem cell transplantation damages cardiac endothelium, which can lead to myocardial necrosis and death.

11. *Answer:* C
    Rationale: Paclitaxel is associated with an asymptomatic bradycardia. Daunorubicin is a DNA intercalator and thus is associated with cardiomyopathy.

12. *Answer:* B
    Rationale: Subacute toxicities occur within 4 to 5 weeks after therapy and are usually reversible. Acute changes occur within 24 hours of drug administration. Chronic changes are not reversible.

13. *Answer:* A
    Rationale: Anthracycline-related cardiotoxicity occurs in up to 40% of clients depending on the cumulative dose of anthracycline administered.

14. *Answer:* A
    Rationale: Although a history of smoking and old age are associated with an increased risk of cardiotoxicity, standard-dose cyclophosphamide, bone metastases, and lung and breast cancer are not.

15. *Answer:* B
    Rationale: The elderly are at greater risk for cardiotoxicity because of slower tissue repair mechanisms and preexisting cardiac disease. Clients with melanoma and women with breast cancer are at high risk of cardiac toxicity related to chemotherapy regimens used to treat their respective diseases.

16. *Answer:* A
    Rationale: High doses of drug administered quickly expose tissues to high levels of agents,

thus increasing risk of toxicity. Lower doses of drugs and 24-hour infusions are not as strongly associated with cardiotoxicity.

17. *Answer:* D
Rationale: Determination of adequate heart functioning should always be accomplished before administration of cardiotoxic chemotherapy. Ejection fraction and cumulative doses should be assessed before administration of DNA intercalators, and electrocardiogram results should be obtained when clients receive agents that interfere with conduction (i.e., paclitaxel).

18. *Answer:* C
Rationale: Potassium and calcium, when abnormal, are associated with muscle weakness and cramping, cardiac abnormalities, and cardiac arrest.

19. *Answer:* B
Rationale: During heart failure, cardiac output decreases, thus causing hematologic congestion in the lungs and neck veins because cardiac output cannot equal venous return to the heart.

20. *Answer:* A
Rationale: Clients with cardiac toxicities may experience discomfort with acute cardiac ischemia but can expect that pain will be controlled. Dyspnea and shortness of breath should be controlled, and education regarding energy conservation should allow the client to maintain normal daily activities.

21. *Answer:* C
Rationale: With additional doses, after a total doxorubicin dosage of 550 mg/m^2 has been reached, the risk of congestive heart failure rises exponentially.

22. *Answer:* C
Rationale: Exercise strengthens cardiac muscle, thus increasing function. Dexrazoxane protects cardiac muscle against the effects of doxorubicin.

23. *Answer:* A
Rationale: Client education is a vital intervention related to cardiotoxicity, since many clients can manage activity well if given the proper education.

24. *Answer:* B
Rationale: Risk of congestive heart failure increases as ejection fraction decreases because the cardiac output cannot keep up with the venous input. Electrocardiograms monitor conductivity, not function. Clients with congestive heart failure are at risk for fluid overload. Fluids should be carefully monitored in these clients.

25. *Answer:* B
Rationale: Lymphedema is the abnormal collection of lymph fluid; hematoma is an abnormal collection of blood in tissues; and hepatoma is a type of malignant liver tumor.

26. *Answer:* C
Rationale: Extracellular fluids are separated by semipermeable membranes surrounding capillaries and cells into interstitial and intravascular components. Normally, more fluid moves from intravascular to interstitial spaces than is returned by the capillary system. The lymphatics remove excess fluid and protein, thus normalizing the fluid balance.

27. *Answer:* D
Rationale: Any factor interfering with the balance of fluid flow, whether lymph or vascular obstruction, can result in edema.

28. *Answer:* D
Rationale: Lack of protein in the body, such as that caused by excessive protein loss or lack of dietary protein intake, alters the fluid balance, allowing excess fluid into the interstitial tissues, resulting in edema.

29. *Answer:* A
Rationale: Mechanical obstruction by tumor or internal venous obstruction by thrombophlebitis changes the pressure gradient so that fluid remains in peripheral tissues.

30. *Answer:* C
Rationale: Dietary factors are considered lifestyle changes over which clients have some control.

31. *Answer:* D
Rationale: All of the answers are objective findings related to malignant edema.

32. *Answer:* C
Rationale: Breast, lung, and hematologic cancers are most commonly associated with malignant pericardial effusions. It may be difficult to assess because most cases are asymptomatic; when they become symptomatic, they are life threatening.

33. *Answer:* A
Rationale: Tumors of the breast, colon, and ovary, for example, that metastasize to the abdominal cavity seed the peritoneum.

34. *Answer:* C
Rationale: Urination is frequent when bladder capacity decreases with additional abdominal fluid. Constipation occurs when motility and capacity are affected by ascites. Shortness of breath is caused by limitation of diaphragmatic movement.

35. *Answer:* B
Rationale: Fluid collection in the lower extremities is associated with malignant edema. Mitomycin C is associated with hemolytic anemia, not thrombotic events. Paraneoplastic syndromes are associated with microangiopathic hemolytic anemia and thrombocytosis.

36. *Answer:* B
Rationale: Bruising and visible blood in the stool are objective signs of bleeding. Severe anemia, thrombocytosis, and abnormal venograms are all testing options that can indicate thrombotic difficulties related to cancer.

BIBLIOGRAPHY

Baker, A.R., & Weber, J.S. (1993). Malignant ascites. In V.T. DeVita, S. Hellman, & S.A. Rosenberg (eds.). *Cancer: Principles and Practices of Oncology* (4th ed.). Philadelphia: JB Lippincott, pp. 2255–2261.

Bunn, P.A., & Ridgeway, E.C. (1993). Paraneoplastic syndromes. In V.T. DeVita, S. Hellman, & S.A. Rosenberg (eds.). *Cancer: Principles and Practices of Oncology* (4th ed.). Philadelphia: JB Lippincott, pp. 2026, 2071.

Ewer, E.S., & Benjamin, R.S. (1997). The cardiotoxicity of chemotherapeutic drugs. In M.C. Perry (ed.). *The Chemotherapy Source Book.* Baltimore: Williams & Wilkins, pp. 582–597.

Gobel, B.H. (1997). Bleeding disorders. In S. Groenwald, M. Frogge, B. Goodman, & C. Yarbro (eds.). *Cancer Nursing: Principles and Practice* (3rd ed.). Boston: Jones & Bartlett, pp. 575–607.

Itano, J., & Taoka, K. (eds.). (1997). *ONS Core Curriculum for Oncology Nursing* (3rd ed.). Philadelphia: WB Saunders, pp. 297–312.

Mrozek-Orlowski, M. (1996). Breast cancer. In M. Liebman & D. Camp-Sorrell (eds.). *Multimodal Therapy in Oncology Nursing.* St. Louis: Mosby, pp. 119–132.

Pass, H.I. (1993). Treatment of malignant pleural and pericardial effusions. In V.T. DeVita, S. Hellman, & S.A. Rosenberg (eds.). *Cancer: Principles and Practices of Oncology* (4th ed.). Philadelphia: JB Lippincott, pp. 2246–2255.

Powel, L. (1996). *Cancer Chemotherapy Guidelines and Recommendations for Practice.* Pittsburgh: Oncology Nursing Press, pp. 12–13.

PART V

Oncologic Emergencies

17

Metabolic Emergencies

Joanne Peter Finley

Select the best answer for each of the following questions:

1. Disseminated intravascular coagulopathy (DIC) is a clotting disorder frequently seen in which malignancy?
   A. Multiple myeloma.
   B. Breast cancer.
   C. Leukemia.
   D. Ovarian cancer.

2. Which condition, other than cancer, may precipitate the onset of DIC?
   A. Immobility.
   B. Antibiotic therapy.
   C. Renal failure.
   D. Gram-negative sepsis.

3. A nurse caring for a client with suspected DIC would expect to find which of the following laboratory results?
   A. Decreased platelets, decreased fibrinogen.
   B. Decreased platelets, increased fibrinogen.
   C. Increased platelets, decreased fibrinogen.
   D. Increased platelets, increased fibrinogen.

4. DIC represents an imbalance of normal coagulation. Which of the following statements best summarizes the characteristics of this condition?
   A. Excessive amounts of clotting factors.
   B. Accelerated coagulation and the formation of excessive thrombin.
   C. Failure of the fibrinolytic system.
   D. Blocked internal pathway of clotting.

5. An abnormal laboratory value associated with DIC is
   A. decreased D-dimers level.
   B. increased platelet count.
   C. elevated fibrin split products.
   D. decreased PTT.

6. The management of DIC includes all of the following treatments *except*
   A. blood component therapy.
   B. chemotherapy.
   C. heparin therapy.
   D. hyperbaric therapy.

7. When assessing the client for DIC, the nurse should be particularly concerned about
   A. mottled extremities.
   B. decreased bowel sounds.
   C. elevated specific gravity.
   D. bradycardia.

8. Nursing care for the client with hypercalcemia should include which of the following measures?
   A. Providing a high-protein, low-salt diet.
   B. Limiting mobility, providing a high-calorie diet.
   C. Increasing hydration, increasing mobility.
   D. Limiting fluid intake, monitoring output.

9. A sign or symptom of hypercalcemia is
   A. diarrhea.
   B. hyperreflexia.
   C. confusion.
   D. oliguria.

10. Serum calcium is decreased by
   A. increased gastrointestinal absorption of calcium.
   B. increased urinary excretion of calcium.
   C. increased levels of parathyroid hormone.
   D. decreased levels of calcitonin.

11. Increased bone resorption in oncology clients is due to all of the following *except*
   A. increased osteoclast activity.
   B. direct tumor invasion of the bone.
   C. increased prostaglandin secretion.
   D. improved mobility.

12. An important nursing consideration when administering gallium nitrate is to
   A. evaluate renal function studies.
   B. monitor blood pressure.
   C. use extravasation precautions.
   D. assess for signs of hyperglycemia.

13. The client most at risk for development of hypercalcemia has a diagnosis of
   A. leukemia.
   B. glioblastoma.
   C. ovarian cancer.
   D. multiple myeloma.

14. J. D. is a 59-year-old woman with breast cancer. Her serum calcium is 12.5 mg/dl. She is alert and oriented with good urine output. The most appropriate intervention to aid in decreasing the serum calcium concentration is to
   A. perform active range of motion exercises.
   B. order a footboard.
   C. ambulate with her.
   D. assist her to stand at the bedside.

15. Signs and symptoms related to syndrome of inappropriate antidiuretic hormone (SIADH) include all of the following *except*
   A. serum hyponatremia.
   B. constipation.
   C. fluid retention.
   D. headache.

16. SIADH is associated with all of the following diseases or treatments *except*
   A. uterine cancer.
   B. vincristine.
   C. small cell lung cancer.
   D. cyclophosphamide.

17. The following are all appropriate interventions for clients with SIADH *except*
   A. forcing fluids.
   B. teaching clients signs and symptoms of hyponatremia.
   C. administering hypertonic saline solution.
   D. restricting fluids.

18. A 26-year-old disoriented and irritable man with Hodgkin's disease and diabetes is admitted to the hospital. His temperature is 100°F, pulse 110, blood pressure 90/40, respiratory rate 30, WBC 500, platelets 150,000. Urine output is normal and positive for sugar (blood sugar is 190). Which condition would you most likely suspect in this client?
   A. Hypocalcemia.
   B. Disseminated intravascular coagulation.
   C. Septic shock.
   D. Diabetic shock.

19. Which absolute granulocyte count places a cancer client at the greatest risk for developing septic shock?
   A. Greater than 1000.
   B. Less than 500.
   C. Greater than 500.
   D. Less than 2500.

20. Septic shock is differentiated from sepsis by which of the following parameters?
   A. Hypotension.
   B. Tachycardia.
   C. Fever.
   D. Tachypnea.

21. The most common cause of sepsis is
   A. viruses.
   B. gram-negative bacteria.
   C. fungi.
   D. gram-positive bacteria.

22. Early interventions in septic shock include
   A. antiendotoxin therapy, IV fluids, hemodynamic monitoring.
   B. IV fluids, hemodynamic monitoring, dopamine.
   C. IV fluids, hemodynamic monitoring, antibiotics.
   D. nutritional support, IV fluids, hemodynamic monitoring.

23. Tumor lysis syndrome occurs most commonly in persons with which cancer?
    A. Renal cell carcinoma.
    B. Breast cancer.
    C. Pancreatic cancer.
    D. High-grade lymphoma.

24. Clients experiencing tumor lysis syndrome may present with which abnormal parameter?
    A. Hypokalemia.
    B. Hypernatremia.
    C. Hypercalcemia.
    D. Hyperkalemia.

25. A 38-year-old man with diffuse histiocytic lymphoma is admitted to the hospital on day 2 of the first cycle of proMACE-CytaBOM chemotherapy. The client complains of weakness, muscle cramps, nausea and vomiting, diarrhea, and oliguria. Laboratory findings are creatinine 2.2, BUN 66, calcium 6.0, phosphorus 8, potassium 5.5, and uric acid 11. ECG changes are evident since last admission. Based on these findings, this client is most likely experiencing which oncologic emergency?
    A. Disseminated intravascular coagulation.
    B. Syndrome of inappropriate antidiuretic hormone.
    C. Tumor lysis syndrome.
    D. Cardiac tamponade.

26. Tumor lysis syndrome (TLS) is a complication of cancer therapy. TLS occurs most commonly in tumors that are
    A. large and rapidly dividing.
    B. slow growing and radiosensitive.
    C. slow growing and chemosensitive.
    D. small and rapidly dividing.

27. A possible complication of tumor lysis syndrome is
    A. adult respiratory distress syndrome.
    B. acute renal failure.
    C. hypokalemia.
    D. bowel obstruction.

28. A client with recurrent ovarian carcinoma has agreed to participate in a clinical trial involving a new agent with anaphylactic potential. What precautions should the nurse take the first time the drug is given?
    A. Premedicate the client with diazepam.
    B. Reject the client as a candidate for the study.
    C. Take vital signs before agent administration and every 4 hours thereafter.
    D. Administer the agent only in an environment where emergency drugs and equipment are readily available.

29. The client's risk for anaphylaxis increases when agents are
    A. given at low doses.
    B. given intravenously.
    C. synthetically prepared.
    D. given as a single dose.

30. Client teaching to decrease the risk of anaphylaxis should include all *except* which of the following?
    A. Signs and symptoms to report to the health care team.
    B. Maintain emergency kit in appropriate place.
    C. Wear Medic Alert jewelry if client has a history of drug allergy.
    D. Administration of oxygen.

ANSWERS

1. *Answer:* C
Rationale: DIC is most frequently associated with promyelocytic leukemia but may occur with any acute leukemia because of the incidence of infection and sepsis. Multiple myeloma, breast cancer, and ovarian cancer do not carry a high incidence of DIC.

2. *Answer:* D
Rationale: Gram-negative sepsis is recognized as a common cause of DIC because of the activation of the intrinsic pathway by endotoxin. Responses A, B, and C are not associated with a high risk of DIC because they do not trigger the coagulation cascade.

3. *Answer:* A
Rationale: Platelet count is decreased as a result of platelet consumption. Plasma fibrinogen is decreased as a result of consumption of fibrinogen by the clotting cascade and by fibrinolysis.

4. *Answer:* B
Rationale: The pathophysiology of DIC involves extensive triggering of the coagulation system, which results in abnormal activation of thrombin formation. Clotting factors are depleted. Fibrinolysis and the clotting pathways continue at a rapid rate.

5. *Answer:* C
Rationale: Elevated fibrin split products are a key diagnostic finding in DIC. The D-dimers and PTT are usually increased, and platelets are decreased in DIC.

6. *Answer:* D
Rationale: Management of DIC includes replacement of blood components lost because of hemorrhage, chemotherapy to treat the underlying cause, and anticoagulants to halt the accelerated coagulation. Hyperbaric therapy has no purpose in DIC management.

7. *Answer:* A
Rationale: Acral cyanosis, or mottled extremities, is a hallmark of DIC. Heart rate is usually increased. Specific gravity is not applicable in this condition. Bowel sounds may be decreased but are not a specific sign.

8. *Answer:* C
Rationale: Increasing hydration will decrease serum calcium by increasing urinary calcium excretion. Improving mobility will decrease serum calcium by decreasing bone resorption. Diet has little bearing on calcium levels in clients with cancer.

9. *Answer:* C
Rationale: Hypercalcemia produces a generalized slowing of functions through neuromuscular depression, i.e., constipation, hyporeflexia, and confusion. Increased urinary calcium usually is manifested in polyuria.

10. *Answer:* B
Rationale: Increased calcium excretion in the urine decreases serum calcium. All of the other measures will increase serum calcium.

11. *Answer:* D
Rationale: Responses A, B, and C all increase bone resorption of calcium and thus increase serum calcium. Improving mobility decreases bone resorption.

12. *Answer:* A
Rationale: Gallium nitrate can impair renal function as evidenced by elevated urea and creatinine levels. Hypotension, extravasation, and hyperglycemia are not seen with gallium nitrate.

13. *Answer:* D
Rationale: There is a 20% to 40% incidence of hypercalcemia in multiple myeloma. Hypercalcemia is not commonly seen in responses A, B, or C.

14. *Answer:* C
Rationale: Although all the interventions help to decrease serum calcium, ambulating the client is the action that will most likely encourage calcium to return to the bone.

15. *Answer:* B
Rationale: Primary symptoms of SIADH are manifestations of water intoxication. Symptoms

listed in responses C and D are attributed to the effects of cerebral edema. Serum hyponatremia is due to the dilutional effect of increased water reabsorption caused by increased levels of ADH. Diarrhea, not constipation, may be seen in SIADH.

16. *Answer:* A
Rationale: Responses B, C, and D are diseases or treatments associated with SIADH. The symptoms of SIADH must be recognized to ensure early detection and appropriate management.

17. *Answer:* A
Rationale: SIADH is essentially manifested by signs of water intoxication. Therefore response A would be inappropriate management.

18. *Answer:* C
Rationale: The signs and symptoms are early manifestations of septic shock. No mention is made of serum calcium or symptoms of hypocalcemia. No mention is made of signs and symptoms of bleeding as seen in DIC. Client's blood sugar is not significantly elevated as in diabetic shock.

19. *Answer:* B
Rationale: An absolute granulocyte count of less than 500 places clients at a higher risk for infection, which may progress to septic shock.

20. *Answer:* A
Rationale: Septic shock is differentiated by hemodynamic instability. Tachycardia, fever, and tachypnea can be seen in sepsis, also.

21. *Answer:* B
Rationale: Gram-negative bacteria are the most common cause of sepsis. Other organisms also may cause sepsis.

22. *Answer:* C
Rationale: Antibiotics on an empiric basis and IV fluids to increase intravascular volume with concurrent hemodynamic monitoring are early interventions. Antiendotoxin therapy is experimental, not a first-line therapy. Nutritional support is important but is not a first intervention. Dopamine is used if IV fluids fail to raise blood pressure.

23. *Answer:* D
Rationale: Persons who have a rapidly divid-

ing cancer are at risk for the development of tumor lysis syndrome because of the large number of cells lysed during therapy. Renal, breast, and pancreatic cancers are not rapidly dividing cancers, and tumor lysis syndrome is rare in clients with solid tumors.

24. *Answer:* D
Rationale: When cells are lysed, potassium is released into the bloodstream, causing abnormally high levels of potassium. Sodium and calcium are not intracellular components and therefore are not released from the cells into the bloodstream. Hypocalcemia actually results because of the binding of calcium to phosphorus.

25. *Answer:* C
Rationale: The client presents with a malignancy that has a high tumor burden and is on day 2 of his chemotherapy cycle. The chemotherapy is causing massive cell lysis, resulting in laboratory values and signs and symptoms consistent with tumor lysis syndrome. There are no signs of bleeding (DIC). No sodium or osmolality levels are reported to determine SIADH. No evidence of cardiac tamponade, i.e., chest pain, dyspnea, muffled heart sounds.

26. *Answer:* A
Rationale: Tumor lysis syndrome most frequently occurs after chemotherapy administration in cancers with a rapidly dividing, large tumor burden.

27. *Answer:* B
Rationale: Acute renal failure is associated with tumor lysis syndrome because of the precipitation in the kidneys of uric acid and calcium phosphate salts. Bowel obstruction and ARDS are not seen with tumor lysis syndrome. Hyperkalemia, not hypokalemia, is associated with it.

28. *Answer:* D
Rationale: Because an anaphylactic reaction may be a life-threatening emergency, appropriate emergency equipment and drugs should be readily available. Diazepam is not a normal premedication. Since every agent has anaphylactic potential, clients are not rejected for studies for this reason alone. Premedications may be given as a precautionary measure. Vital signs usually are taken more often for a drug with anaphylactic potential, especially during the first hour.

29. *Answer:* B

Rationale: Intravenous administration of drugs increases the risk for anaphylaxis because of the rapid, systemic effect. Other factors associated with an increased risk of anaphylaxis are high dosages, naturally occurring agents, and intermittent administration (which delays the antibody formation to the antigen).

30. *Answer:* D

Rationale: Administration of oxygen does not decrease the *risk* of anaphylaxis. Clients' knowledge of signs and symptoms to report will allow them to alert health personnel for early interventions to be instituted. Emergency kits also need to be available for immediate interventions. Medic Alert jewelry may prevent anaphylaxis by making others aware of a known allergy.

BIBLIOGRAPHY

Arrambide, K., & Toto, R.D. (1993). Tumor lysis syndrome. *Semin Nephrol 13*(3), 273–280.

Batcheller, J. (1994). Syndrome of inappropriate antidiuretic hormone secretion. *Crit Care Nurs Clin North Am 6*(4), 687–692.

Bick, R.L. (1994). Disseminated intravascular coagulation. Objective criteria for diagnosis and management. *Med Clin North Am 78*(3), 511–543.

Bone, R.C. (1994). Sepsis and its complications: The clinical problem. *Crit Care Med 22*(7), S8–S12.

Bunn, P.A., & Ridgway, E.C. (1993). Paraneoplastic syndromes. In V.T. DeVita, S. Hellman, & S.A. Rosenberg (eds.). *Cancer: Principles and Practice of Oncology* (4th ed.). Philadelphia: JB Lippincott.

Cordisco, M.E. (1994). Fighting DIC. *RN 57*(8), 36–40.

Ferguson, K.L., & Brown, L. (1996). Bacteremia and sepsis. *Emerg Med Clin North Am 14*(1), 185–194.

Hawthorne, J.L., Schneider, S.M., & Workman, M.L. (1992). Common electrolyte imbalances associated with malignancy. *AACN Clin Issues Crit Care Nurs 3*(3), 714–723.

Kurtz, A. (1993). Disseminated intravascular coagulation with leukemia patients. *Cancer Nurs 16*(6), 456–463.

McCoy-Adabody, A.M., & Borger, D.L. (1996). Selected critical care complications of cancer therapy. *AACN Clin Issues 7*(1), 26–36.

Singer, F.R., & Minoofar, P.N. (1995). Biphosphonates in the treatment of disorders of mineral metabolism. *Adv Endocrinol Metab 6*, 259–288.

Sriskandan, S., & Cohen, J. (1995). The pathogenesis of septic shock. *J Infect 30*, 201–206.

Yucha, C.B., & Toto, K.H. (1994). Calcium and phosphorus derangements. *Crit Care Nurs Clin North Am 6*(4), 747–759.

NOTES

18

Structural Emergencies

Jane C. Hunter and Marilyn A. Kline

Select the best answer for each of the following questions:

1. What is the most accurate diagnostic test for cardiac tamponade?
   - A. CT scan.
   - B. Chest x-ray.
   - C. Echocardiogram.
   - D. ECG.

2. An individual with which cancer is at risk for developing cardiac tamponade?
   - A. Lung cancer.
   - B. Sarcoma.
   - C. Hodgkin's disease.
   - D. Colon cancer.

3. All of the following signs and symptoms are seen in cardiac tamponade *except*
   - A. dyspnea.
   - B. cough.
   - C. narrowing pulse pressure.
   - D. bradycardia.

4. All of the following represent signs and symptoms of cardiac tamponade *except*
   - A. retrosternal chest pain.
   - B. muffled heart sounds.
   - C. increased jugular vein distention.
   - D. widening pulse pressure.

5. All of the following pharmaceutical interventions have been used for pericardial sclerosis *except*
   - A. tetracycline.
   - B. thiotepa.

   - C. vincristine.
   - D. nitrogen mustard.

6. Which cancer does not place an individual at high risk of spinal cord compression?
   - A. Brain.
   - B. Lung.
   - C. Breast.
   - D. Prostate.

7. All of the following interventions may be used in the treatment of spinal cord compression *except*
   - A. steroids.
   - B. radiation therapy.
   - C. biologic response agents.
   - D. laminectomy.

8. The most common symptom of early spinal cord compression is
   - A. motor weakness.
   - B. sensory loss.
   - C. sexual impotence.
   - D. back pain.

9. All of the following interventions are indicated in monitoring for progression of spinal cord compression *except*
   - A. palpation of the bladder.
   - B. assessment for increased severity of pain.
   - C. observation for peripheral edema.
   - D. assessment for decreased coordination.

10. All of the following interventions are important in planning home care for clients with spinal cord compression *except*

A. helping the client and family focus on realistic goals to maintain independence.
B. collaborating with physical therapy in the evaluation of assistive devices.
C. consulting a social worker to identify community resources and support groups.
D. teaching the client and family to avoid blood pressure measurement and venipuncture in upper extremities.

11. The malignancy associated with superior vena cava syndrome (SVCS) most frequently is
   A. germ cell tumor.
   B. lymphoma.
   C. breast cancer.
   D. lung cancer.

12. Interventions for the management of superior vena cava syndrome (SVCS) include all of the following *except*
   A. reassuring that physical appearance will return to normal as SVCS resolves.
   B. monitoring blood pressure every hour in unaffected arm.
   C. administering O_2 by nasal cannula at 2 L/min.
   D. elevating head of bed to 60 degrees.

13. Individuals with which of the following cancers are at high risk for SVCS?
   A. Lymphoma/lung.
   B. Liver/lymphoma.
   C. Breast/cervical.
   D. Genitourinary/gastrointestinal.

14. What is the single most important sequela that indicates the increasing severity of SVCS?
   A. Progressive dyspnea.
   B. Visual disturbances.
   C. Irritability.
   D. Chronic headaches.

15. Which of the following is *not* an early sign of SVCS?
   A. Nonproductive cough.
   B. Dyspnea.

C. Blurred vision.
D. Hoarseness.

16. Persons with which of the following cancers are *not* at risk for developing increased intracranial pressure?
   A. Lung cancer.
   B. Melanoma.
   C. Breast cancer.
   D. Multiple myeloma.

17. Systemic chemotherapy is *least* effective in which structural oncologic emergency?
   A. Increased intracranial pressure.
   B. Superior vena cava syndrome.
   C. Cardiac tamponade.
   D. Spinal cord compression.

18. Which of the following signs and symptoms indicate increased intracranial pressure?
   A. Normal blood pressure.
   B. Agitation.
   C. Narrowing pulse pressure.
   D. Widening pulse pressure.

19. Which of the following interventions decreases the severity of symptoms associated with increased intracranial pressure?
   A. Instructing the client to avoid the Valsalva maneuver.
   B. Keeping the client supine.
   C. Encouraging the client to cough frequently.
   D. Administering furosemide.

20. Which mechanisms are responsible for an increase in intracranial pressure in clients with cancer?
   A. Tumor size and papilledema.
   B. Tumor size and peripheral edema.
   C. Tumor size and cerebral edema.
   D. Tumor type and grade.

ANSWERS

1. *Answer:* C
Rationale: Echocardiogram is an accurate, noninvasive method to determine pericardial effusion. It can be done quickly and can even be done at the bedside if necessary.

2. *Answer:* A
Rationale: Lung cancer, breast cancer, leukemia, and non-Hodgkin's lymphoma are among common cancers that can metastasize to the heart.

3. *Answer:* D
Rationale: Bradycardia is not associated with cardiac tamponade.

4. *Answer:* D
Rationale: In cardiac tamponade there is a narrowing of the pulse pressure, which is indicated by a decreased systolic and increased diastolic blood pressure.

5. *Answer:* C
Rationale: Tetracycline, nitrogen mustard, and thiotepa have been used as sclerosing agents.

6. *Answer:* A
Rationale: Cancers of the breast, lung, and prostate have a natural history of metastases to vertebral bodies, which may compress the cord.

7. *Answer:* C
Rationale: Biological response agents are not indicated to treat spinal cord compression. Radiation therapy may be used alone or in combination with surgery. Steroids may be given to reduce spinal cord edema and pain. Decompression by laminectomy or resection of a vertebral body is used as treatment for spinal cord compression if the tumor is not responsive to radiation therapy or if the disease recurs in an area already treated with radiation therapy.

8. *Answer:* D
Rationale: When tumors press on the spinal cord, pain is usually the initial complaint. The other options are late symptoms.

9. *Answer:* C
Rationale: Peripheral edema is not a progressive motor neurologic deficit that can be caused by spinal cord compression.

10. *Answer:* D
Rationale: Assisting clients to maintain independence with appropriate use of resources is an important goal of nursing care.

11. *Answer:* D
Rationale: Lung cancer is most frequently associated with superior vena cava syndrome (SVCS). Clients with lymphoma of the mediastinum, germ cell tumors, breast cancer, and Kaposi's sarcoma are also at risk for SVCS.

12. *Answer:* B
Rationale: Procedures that cause constriction in the upper extremities should be avoided because venous return is already compromised in SVCS. Instead, blood pressure should be monitored on the thigh.

13. *Answer:* A
Rationale: Clients with a diagnosis of lymphoma of the mediastinum and lung cancer are at risk for SVCS.

14. *Answer:* A
Rationale: Progressive dyspnea, indicating airway obstruction, can result in respiratory arrest and death.

15. *Answer:* C
Rationale: Blurred vision is a sequela of intracranial hypertension and is not a presenting symptom of SVCS.

16. *Answer:* D
Rationale: Tumor cells from breast and lung cancer and melanoma often metastasize to the brain.

17. *Answer:* A
Rationale: Most chemotherapy agents do not cross the blood-brain barrier to kill cancer cells. Chemotherapy has known efficacy, either alone or in combination with other treatment modalities in SVCS, cardiac tamponade, and spinal cord compression.

18. *Answer:* D

Rationale: Among the late signs of increased intracranial pressure are an increase in systolic blood pressure and a decrease in the diastolic blood pressure, which indicates a widening pulse pressure.

19. *Answer:* A

Rationale: All responses except the Valsalva maneuver do not change the severity of symptoms associated with increased intracranial pressure.

20. *Answer:* C

Rationale: The size of the tumor and the presence of cerebral edema compete for space within the skull, resulting in increased intracranial pressure.

BIBLIOGRAPHY

Clezki, J., & Macklis, R.M. (1995). The palliative role of radiotherapy in the management of the cancer patient. *Semin Oncol 22*(2[suppl 3]), 82–90.

Davies, P.S. (1995). Neoplastic cardiac tamponade. In C. Miaskowski & K.V. Gettrust (eds.). *Oncology Nursing: Plans and Care for Specialty Practice.* Albany: Delmar Publishers, pp. 279–285.

Dunne-Daly, C.F. (1994). Radiation therapy for oncologic emergencies. *Cancer Nurs 17*(6), 516–527.

Gates, M.L. (1995). Superior vena cava syndrome. In C. Miaskowski & K.V. Gettrust (eds.). *Oncology Nursing: Plans and Care for Specialty Practice.* Albany: Delmar Publishers, pp. 315–323.

Hunter, J.C. (1998). Structural emergencies. In J.K. Itano & K.N. Taoka (eds.). *Core Curriculum for Oncology Nursing* (3rd ed.). Philadelphia: WB Saunders, pp. 340–354.

Kazierad, D. (1998). Obstructive emergencies, increased intracranial pressure. In B.L. Johnson & J. Gross (eds.). *Handbook of Oncology Nursing* (3rd ed.). Boston: Jones & Bartlett, pp. 617–631.

Kazierad, D. (1998). Obstructive emergencies, spinal cord compression. In B.L. Johnson & J. Gross (eds.). *Handbook of Oncology Nursing* (3rd ed.). Boston: Jones & Bartlett, pp. 631–644.

Kilbride, S.S. (1998). Obstructive emergencies, cardiac tamponade. In B.L. Johnson & J. Gross (eds.). *Handbook of Oncology Nursing* (3rd ed.). Boston: Jones & Bartlett, pp. 673–686.

Kreamer, K. (1998). Obstructive emergencies, superior vena cava syndrome. In B.L. Johnson & J. Gross (eds.). *Handbook of Oncology Nursing* (3rd ed.). Boston: Jones & Bartlett, pp. 645–654.

Maxwell, M. (1997). Malignant effusions and edemas. In S. Groenwald, M.H. Frogge, M. Goodman, & C.H. Yarbro (eds.). *Cancer Nursing: Principles and Practice.* Boston: Jones & Bartlett, pp. 721–741.

NOTES

PART VI

Scientific Basis for Practice

19

Carcinogenesis

Deborah Lowe Volker

Select the best answer for each of the following questions:

1. Failure of systemic therapy for cancer is best explained by the tumor property of
   A. heterogeneity.
   B. anaplasia.
   C. necrosis.
   D. metastasis.

2. Specific tumors tend to metastasize to specific target organs because
   A. the immune system selectively destroys metastatic deposits to nontarget organs.
   B. therapeutic levels of chemotherapy may not be achieved in target organs.
   C. target organs are more vascular, thus providing more nutrients to metastatic cells.
   D. metastatic cells may be able to elicit necessary growth factors only in target organs.

3. The tumor grade refers to the
   A. expression of tumor-associated antigens.
   B. degree of differentiation of malignant cells.
   C. extent of chromosomal aberrations.
   D. likelihood of metastatic spread.

4. According to the TNM staging system, which of the following is indicative of highly advanced disease?
   A. T1 N1 M0.
   B. T3 N0 M0.
   C. T3 N3 M1.
   D. T2 N1 M1.

5. Which of the following histologic conditions is most strongly associated with malignancy?
   A. Hyperplasia.
   B. Metaplasia.
   C. Anaplasia.
   D. Dysplasia.

ANSWERS

1. *Answer:* A

   Rationale: Although all of the options describe properties of malignant tumors, the problem of heterogeneity best answers the question because it refers to the marked variations between individual cells within a tumor. These variations cause the tumor to have varying susceptibilities to treatment.

2. *Answer:* D

   Rationale: Although there are many hypotheses to explain the organ specificity of metastasis, response D is the only choice of the four that is currently supported by experimental studies.

3. *Answer:* B

   Rationale: Tumor grading refers to the degree of differentiation of the malignant cells. The other three choices describe properties of many cancers.

4. *Answer:* C

   Rationale: Of the four, option C denotes the greatest amount of disease. C indicates more advanced disease than both A and B because C has metastatic involvement. Although both C and D contain metastatic involvement, C has larger tumor and more nodal involvement.

5. *Answer:* C

   Rationale: Hyperplasia, metaplasia, and dysplasia are not neoplastic but may precede the development of cancer. Anaplasia, the hallmark of malignancy, refers to the most poorly differentiated cells that occur in deranged growth patterns.

BIBLIOGRAPHY

Caudell, K., Cuaron, L., & Gallucci, B. (1996). Cancer biology: Molecular and cellular aspects. In R. McCorkle, M. Grant, M. Frank-Stromborg, & S. Baird (eds.). *Cancer Nursing: A Comprehensive Textbook* (2nd ed.). Philadelphia: WB Saunders, pp. 150–170.

Mettlin, C., & Michalek, A. (1996). The causes of cancer. In R. McCorkle, M. Grant, M. Frank-Stromborg, & S. Baird (eds.). *Cancer Nursing: A Comprehensive Textbook* (2nd ed.). Philadelphia: WB Saunders, pp. 138–149.

Pamies, R.J., & Crawford, D.T. (1996). Tumor markers: An update. *Med Clin North Am 80*(1), 185–199.

Soltis, M., Hubbard, S., & Kohn, E. (1996). The biology of invasion and metastases. In R. McCorkle, M. Grant, M. Frank-Stromborg, & S. Baird (eds.). *Cancer Nursing: A Comprehensive Textbook* (2nd ed.). Philadelphia: WB Saunders, pp. 190–212.

Volker, D.L. (1998). Carcinogenesis. In J. Itano & K. Taoka (eds.). *Core Curriculum for Oncology Nursing* (3rd ed.). Philadelphia: WB Saunders, pp. 357–382.

20

Immunology

Lynne Brophy

Select the best answer for each of the following questions:

1. Which of the following is *not* one of the four functions of the immune system?
   - A. Protection.
   - B. Surveillance.
   - C. Homeostasis.
   - D. Repair.

2. Which of the following cells often destroy pathogens that enter the tissues?
   - A. T cells.
   - B. Monocytes.
   - C. Phagocytes.
   - D. Tissue macrophages.

3. Which of the following is not a function of acquired immunity?
   - A. Recognition and destruction of antigens.
   - B. Production of specialized antibodies.

   - C. Lysis of foreign cells.
   - D. Initiation of the inflammation process.

4. Which phrase best describes the functions of cytokines?
   - A. Communicate messages from cell to cell.
   - B. Stimulate growth differentiation.
   - C. Regulate the neuroendocrine system.
   - D. Guard against invading pathogens.

5. Which conditions that are often present in persons with cancer are thought to affect the immune response?
   - A. Advanced age, immunosuppression, and a history of skin cancer.
   - B. Advanced age, immunosuppression, and a history of alcoholism.
   - C. Immunosuppression, malnourishment, and a history of chronic illness.
   - D. Obesity, immunosuppression, advanced age, and a history of extreme stress.

ANSWERS

1. *Answer:* D

    Rationale: The immune system is an integrated network that has four functions: protection, surveillance, homeostasis, and regulation of immune responses.

2. *Answer:* D

    Rationale: Nonmobile macrophages, which exist in the tissues, begin phagocytizing a foreign body after it has invaded the tissues.

3. *Answer:* D

    Rationale: Recognition and destruction of antigens, production of specialized antibodies, and lysis of foreign cells are all functions of acquired or specific immunity. The inflammation process provides nonspecific defense against foreign invaders.

4. *Answer:* A

    Rationale: Cytokines are proteins produced by cells that secrete substances which communicate messages to other *cells.* Examples of cytokines include interleukins, interferons, lymphokines, and monokines.

5. *Answer:* C

    Rationale: When an individual is malnourished, elderly, chronically ill, immunosuppressed or under significant stress, the immune system can fail to recognize and destroy abnormal or foreign cells, and cancer may develop.

BIBLIOGRAPHY

Gallucci, B., & McCarthy, D. (1995). The immune system. In P. Trahan Reiger (ed.). *Biotherapy: A Comprehensive Nursing Overview.* Boston: Jones & Bartlett, pp. 15–42.

Guyton, A.C., & Hall, J.E. (1997). *Human Physiology and Mechanisms of Disease* (6th ed.). Philadelphia: WB Saunders.

Kuby, J. (1992). *Immunology.* New York: W.H. Freeman.

Pfeifer, K.A. (1994). Pathophysiology. In S.E. Otto (ed.). *Oncology Nursing* (2nd ed.). St. Louis: Mosby, pp. 3–19.

Sahai, J., & Louie, S.G. (1993). Overview of the immune and hematopoietic systems. *Am J Hosp Pharm 50*(7 Suppl 3), 4–9.

Workman, M.L. (1995). Essential concepts of inflammation and immunity. *Crit Care Nurs Clin North Am 7*(4), 601–615.

Wujcik, D. (1995). Hematopoietic growth factors. In P. Trahan Reiger (ed.). *Biotherapy: A Comprehensive Nursing Overview.* Boston: Jones & Bartlett, pp. 113–133.

21

Genetics

Kathleen A. Calzone

Select the best answer for each of the following questions:

1. A gene is which of the following?
   A. A threadlike structure that contains genetic information.
   B. An individual unit of hereditary information.
   C. A sequence of amino acids.
   D. Two nucleotide chains, running in opposite directions that are coiled around one another to form a double helix.

2. What is a gene with a change in its DNA pattern?
   A. Tumor suppressor gene.
   B. Proto-oncogene.
   C. Mismatch repair gene.
   D. Mutation.

3. One critical component of informed consent for predisposition genetic testing for inherited cancer risk is

   A. confirmation of the family history for cancer.
   B. overview of the risks and benefits of predisposition genetic testing.
   C. recommending an individualized cancer risk management plan before testing should the client be found to harbor an alteration in a cancer susceptibility gene.
   D. completion of a full history and physical to rule out any suspicion of cancer.

4. The primary role of the nurse in predisposition genetic testing includes
   A. establishing a cancer risk management plan.
   B. determining which members of a family should be tested for a genetic alteration.
   C. facilitating informed decision making without being directive.
   D. selecting the laboratory to perform the test.

ANSWERS

1. *Answer:* B

Rationale: Genes are individual units of hereditary information located at a specific position on a chromosome and consist of a sequence of DNA that codes for a specific protein. A threadlike structure that contains genetic information refers to chromosomes. Genes code for a sequence of amino acids resulting in a protein that has a specific function. A double helix refers to DNA (deoxyribonucleic acid).

2. *Answer:* D

Rationale: Mutations are variations in the sequence of DNA. Tumor suppressor genes, proto-oncogenes, and mismatch repair genes are different types of regulatory genes that control cell growth and proliferation. When functioning normally without the presence of a pathologic mutation, all of these genes appear to prevent the development of cancer.

3. *Answer:* B

Rationale: The decision whether to undergo predisposition genetic testing is hinged on the adequacy of the information provided to the individual in regard to the risks and benefits of testing. Confirmation of the family history of cancer is a critical component of determining eligibility for predisposition genetic testing but is not part of the informed consent process. There is insufficient data regarding the benefits and limitations of all cancer risk management strategies in individuals at high risk for cancer because of an alteration in a cancer susceptibility gene. The health care provider should outline the potential alternatives and limitations of cancer risk management as part of the informed consent process but should not recommend a particular strategy. Informed consent for predisposition genetic testing does not depend on the client's personal health status. However, current health status established by a history and physical is an essential component of cancer risk counseling.

4. *Answer:* C

Rationale: The primary role of the nurse in predisposition genetic testing should be to provide the information necessary for an informed decision without being directive in regard to the testing decision. Also, the nurse should be sure that the client understands that testing is completely voluntary and will not prejudice his or her future health care. The nurse should outline the potential alternatives and limitations of cancer risk management as part of the informed consent process but should not recommend a particular strategy. The nurse can play a role in identifying family members who are eligible for testing, but testing is completely voluntary, and no health care provider should dictate who should be tested. In addition, this should not be considered a primary role for the nurse. Laboratories where predisposition genetic testing is performed should be Clinical Laboratory Improvement Act (CLIA) approved. However, the primary role of the nurse is to facilitate informed decision making.

BIBLIOGRAPHY

American Society of Clinical Oncology. (1996). Genetic testing for cancer susceptibility. *J Clin Oncol 14*, 1730–1736.

American Society of Human Genetics. (1996). Statement on informed consent for genetic research. *Am J Hum Genet 59*, 471–474.

Burke, W., Daly, M., Garber, J., Botkin, J., Kahn, M.J.E., Lynch, P., McTiernan, A., Offit, K., Perlman, J., Peterson, G., Thomson, E., Varricchio, C. (1997). Recommendations for follow-up care of individuals with an inherited predisposition to cancer II. BRCA1 and BRCA2. *JAMA 277*, 997–1003.

Burke, W., Peterson, G., Lynch, P., Botkin, J., Daly, M., Garber, J., Kahn, M.J.E., McTiernan, A., Offit, K., Thomson, E., Varricchio, C. (1997). Recommendations for follow-up care of individuals with an inherited predisposition to cancer I. Hereditary non-polyposis colon cancer. *JAMA 277*, 915–919.

Calzone, K.A. (1998). Genetics. In J. Itano & K. Taoka (eds.). *Core Curriculum for Oncology Nursing* (3rd ed.). Philadelphia: WB Saunders, pp. 392–403.

Carter, M. (1995). Patient-provider relationship in the context of genetic testing for hereditary cancers. *J Natl Cancer Inst 17*, 119–121.

Caudell, K.A., Cuaron, L.J., Gallucci, B.B. (1996). Cancer biology: Molecular and cellular aspects. In R. McCorkle, M. Grant, M. Frank-Stromborg, & S.B. Baird (eds.). *Cancer Nursing: A Comprehensive Textbook* (2nd ed.). Philadelphia: WB Saunders, pp. 150–170.

Kelly, P.T. (1992). Informational needs of individuals and families with hereditary cancers. *Semin Oncol Nurs 8*, 288–292.

Lea, D.H., Williams, J., & Tinley, S.T. (1994). Nursing and genetic health care. *J Genet Counsel 3*, 113–124.

Mettlin, C., & Michalek, A.M. (1996). The causes of cancer. In R. McCorkle, M. Grant, M. Frank-Stromborg, & S.B. Baird (eds.). *Cancer Nursing: A Comprehensive Textbook* (2nd ed.). Philadelphia: WB Saunders, pp. 138–149.

Weinberg, R.A. (1994). Oncogenes and tumor suppressor genes. *CA: Cancer J Clin 44*, 160–170.

22

Nursing Care of the Client with Breast Cancer

Marge Bernice

Select the best answer for each of the following questions:

1. Most breast cancers occur in which area of the breast?
   A. Upper outer quadrant.
   B. Upper inner quadrant.
   C. Lower outer quadrant.
   D. Beneath the nipple.

2. After mastectomy, which of the following symptoms should be reported to a health care provider as soon as it is observed?
   A. Numbness of affected arm.
   B. Increase in size of affected arm.
   C. Absence of sensation on the chest wall.
   D. "Phantom breast" sensation.

3. Which of the following is a possible adverse effect of tamoxifen (Nolvadex) therapy?
   A. Ovarian cancer.
   B. Excess vaginal secretions.
   C. Decreased bone density.
   D. Hot flashes.

4. Breast cancer hormone receptor assay test results may be used for all of the following *except*
   A. predicting response to hormonal treatments.
   B. predicting prognosis.
   C. determining if lymph nodes need to be removed.
   D. deciding on adjuvant treatment options.

5. Which of the following statements about breast conservation therapy is *false*?
   A. It is an appropriate method of primary therapy for most women with stage I and II breast cancer.
   B. Breast conservation therapy for invasive breast cancer consists of limited surgery followed by radiation therapy.
   C. The 5-year survival rate is equivalent to mastectomy.
   D. Breast conservation is contraindicated if axillary lymph nodes are positive.

ANSWERS

1. *Answer:* A
   Rationale: Approximately half of malignant tumors occur in the upper outer quadrant of the breast where the largest proportion of breast tissue is located. About 20% are found beneath the nipple; breast cancers occur less frequently in other quadrants of the breast.

2. *Answer:* B
   Rationale: An increase in diameter of the affected arm is a symptom of lymphedema and should be reported immediately. Numbness of the affected arm and chest wall and "phantom breast" are common, expected postoperative sensations.

3. *Answer:* D
   Rationale: Hot flashes and vaginal dryness are common side effects of tamoxifen therapy. There is a slightly increased incidence of endometrial cancer, but no reported increase in ovarian cancer, in women taking tamoxifen. Rather than decreasing bone density, tamoxifen actually protects against bone loss.

4. *Answer:* C
   Rationale: Hormone receptor assay results provide independent prognostic information and predict response to hormonal treatments and therefore can be useful in deciding on systemic treatment options but have no bearing on local treatment decisions such as surgery or lymph node dissection.

5. *Answer:* D
   Rationale: Answers A, B, and C are true. Axillary lymph node involvement is *not* a contraindication to breast conservation therapy.

BIBLIOGRAPHY

Bernice, M., & Entrekin, N. (1998). Nursing care of the client with breast cancer. In J. Itano & K. Taoka (eds.). *Core Curriculum in Oncology Nursing* (3rd ed.). Philadelphia: WB Saunders, pp. 404–420.

Chapman, D.D., & Goodman, M. (1997). Breast cancer. In S.L. Groenwald, M.H. Frogge, M. Goodman, & C.H. Yarbro (eds.). *Cancer Nursing: Principles and Practice* (4th ed.). Boston: Jones & Bartlett, pp. 916–979.

Donegan, W.L., & Spratt, J.S. (eds.). (1995). *Cancer of the Breast* (4th ed.). Philadelphia: WB Saunders.

Dow, K.H. (ed.). (1996). *Contemporary Issues in Breast Cancer.* Boston: Jones & Bartlett.

Engelking, C. (ed.-in-chief) & Kalinowski, B.H. (guest ed.). (1995). *A Comprehensive Guide to Breast Cancer Treatment: Current Issues and Controversies* [monograph]. New York: Triclinica Communications.

Knobf, M.T. (1996). Breast cancers. In R. McCorkle, M. Grant, M. Frank-Stromborg, & S.B. Baird (eds.). *Cancer Nursing: A Comprehensive Textbook* (2nd ed.). Philadelphia: WB Saunders, pp. 547–610.

Leitch, A.M., Dodd, G.D., Costanza, M., Linver, M., Pressman, P., McGinnis, L., & Smith, R.A. (1997). American Cancer Society guidelines for the early detection of breast cancer: Update 1997. *CA 47,* 150–153.

23

Nursing Care of the Client with Cancer of the Urinary System

Julena Lind

Select the best answer for each of the following questions:

1. Which of the following statements best describes the growth and prognosis of renal cell cancer?
   - A. Once the disease has spread to the lymph nodes, the 5-year survival rate is approximately 65% to 70%.
   - B. New advances in the diagnosis and treatment of renal cell cancer have improved 5-year survival by 65% to 70%.
   - C. Renal cell tumors primarily spread to the liver and brain with 5-year survival of 10% to 50%.
   - D. Thirty percent of renal cell cancers are advanced at the time of diagnosis, with 5-year survival of 10% to 50%.

2. Mr. W. has returned home after having had a radical nephrectomy for renal cell cancer and is about to begin treatment with interleukin-2 and alpha interferon. Appropriate *home* nursing interventions for Mr. W. include all of the following *except*
   - A. reminding Mr. W. to schedule a follow-up appointment to monitor HCG and alpha-fetoprotein levels.
   - B. assessing for respiratory function and pain management status.
   - C. ensuring that Mr. W. and his family understand the instructions regarding ac-etaminophen and that they have the medication available at home.
   - D. follow-up teaching on the importance of liberal fluid intake.

3. Nurses should teach clients all of the following American Cancer Society Guidelines for prostate cancer screening *except*
   - A. annual digital rectal examination beginning at age 40.
   - B. transrectal ultrasound annually beginning at age 50.
   - C. prostatic antigen screening at age 50 and each year after.
   - D. prostate examination annually beginning at age 50.

4. Mr. Y. has just been diagnosed with stage B prostate cancer. His treatment options include
   - A. radical prostatectomy, followed by brachytherapy and hormonal therapy.
   - B. brachytherapy followed by chemotherapy and a course of biologic response modifiers.
   - C. radical prostatectomy with lymph node dissection or high dose (6000 to 7000 cGy) external beam radiation therapy.
   - D. external beam radiation therapy followed by hormonal therapy.

5. Side effects after radical prostatectomy include
   - A. incontinence, impotence, and hematuria.
   - B. impotence, myelosuppression, and dysuria.

C. cystitis, urethral strictures, diarrhea, and lower extremity bleeding.

D. hot flashes, decreased libido, and elevated PSA levels.

6. The following all describe nursing care of the client receiving intravesical BCG for bladder cancer *except*

A. the drug should be treated as infectious waste and if given at home, the toilet should be disinfected with undiluted household bleach.

B. a fever above 101°F for 7 days or more is common and should be treated with acetaminophen.

C. Instruct the client that during the first hour after instillation, he or she should lie on his or her stomach, back, and each side for 15 minutes each. This encourages maximum distribution of the drug in the bladder.

D. Urgency, dysuria, and hematuria usually begin after 2 to 3 instillations and increase with the frequency and number of instillations.

NOTES

ANSWERS

1. *Answer:* D

   Rationale: Once the disease has spread, 5-year survival is 50% or less. Renal cell tumors spread to the lymph nodes and the bones. New advances in treatment have not made a dramatic improvement in survival. D is the correct answer because the disease is advanced at diagnosis in approximately one third of all clients and the 5-year survival rate is not high.

2. *Answer:* A

   Rationale: Treatment with interleukin-2 and alpha interferon often causes fever and flulike symptoms that are mitigated by premedication with acetaminophen. Fluids should be encouraged for postnephrectomy clients to promote the health of the remaining kidney. HCG and alpha-fetoprotein levels are laboratory studies that help monitor testicular cancer. Pain and respiratory function are common problems after nephrectomy.

3. *Answer:* B

   Rationale: Transrectal ultrasound is often recommended as a follow-up to an abnormal PSA finding, but is not currently recommended routinely on an annual basis.

4. *Answer:* C

   Rationale: Standard treatment for cure of a tumor confined to the prostate gland (stage B) is radical prostatectomy with lymph node dissection *or* radiation therapy. Hormonal therapy is reserved for advanced disease. Biologic response modifiers are not part of the standard treatment for early prostate cancer.

5. *Answer:* A

   Rationale: The three most frequent side effects of radical prostatectomy are incontinence, impotence, and early postoperative hematuria. Myelopsuppression, cystitis, urethral strictures, diarrhea, lower extremity bleeding, hot flashes, decreased libido, and elevated PSA levels are not common side effects of prostatectomy.

6. *Answer:* B

   Rationale: A fever of above 101°F for more than 7 days is abnormal and should be reported to the physician, because it could indicate a severe inflammatory response.

BIBLIOGRAPHY

Bono, A.V. (1994). Superficial bladder cancer: State of the art. *Cancer Chemother Pharmacol 35*(suppl.), S101–S109.

Chodak, G.W., Thisted, R.A., & Gerber, G.S., et al. (1994). Results of conservative management of clinically localized prostate cancer. *N Engl J Med 330*(4), 242–248.

Davis, M. (1993). Renal cell carcinoma. *Semin Oncol Nurs 9*(4), 267–271.

Hostetler, R.M., Mandel, I.G., & Marshburn, J. (1996). Prostate cancer screening. *Med Clin North Am 80*(1), 83–98.

McLeod, D.G., & Kolvenbag, G.J. (1996). Defining the role of antiandrogens in the treatment of prostate cancer. *Urology 47*(1A), 95–96.

McLeod, D.G., & Moul, J.W. (1995). Controversies in the treatment of prostate cancer with maximal androgen deprivation. *Surg Oncol Clin North Am 4*(2), 345–359.

Mandelson, M.T., Wager, E.H., & Thompson, R.S. (1995). PSA screening: A public health dilemma. *Annu Rev Public Health 16*, 283–306.

Ofman, U.S. (1993). Psychosocial and sexual implications of genitourinary cancers. *Semin Oncol Nurs 9*(4), 286–292.

Razor, B.R. (1993). Continent urinary reservoirs. *Semin Oncol Nurs 9*(4), 272–285.

Taneja, S.S., Pierce, W., Figlin, R., & Belldegrun, A. (1994). Management of disseminated kidney cancer. *Urol Clin North Am 21*(4), 625–637.

Zietman, A.L., Coen, J.J., & Dallow, K.C., et al. (1995). The treatment of prostate cancer by conventional radiation therapy: An analysis of long-term outcome. *Int J Radiat Oncol Biol Phys 32*(2), 287–292.

24

Nursing Care of the Client with Lung Cancer

Julena Lind

Select the best answer for each of the following questions:

1. Which of the following cancers would have the shortest and poorest prognosis?
   A. Extensive small cell lung cancer (SCLC).
   B. Limited small cell lung cancer.
   C. Non-small cell lung cancer (NSCLC) stage I.
   D. Non-small cell lung cancer, stage II.

2. Mrs. B.'s small cell lung cancer has just been diagnosed. Which of the following best describes what the nurse should know to support Mrs. B. and her family during the time just before beginning treatment.
   A. SCLC is usually treated with partial lobectomy to remove the primary tumor followed by intensive chemotherapy.
   B. Radiotherapy alone (i.e., prophylactic cranial irradiation as an adjunct to high-dose brachytherapy) as primary, definitive treatment.
   C. SCLC generally has a better prognosis than non-small cell lung cancer and can be treated less aggressively.
   D. Etoposide and carboplatin are often given for 4 to 6 months to treat SCLC.

3. All of the following are risk factors for lung cancer *except*
   A. having smoked 2 or more packs of cigarettes per day for 10 years or more.
   B. having had long-term intensive exposure to asbestos.
   C. a history of tuberculosis and COPD.
   D. uranium or radon gas exposure especially in smokers.

4. Many clients with lung cancer require symptom management and supportive treatment as part of their nursing care. All of the following are potential nursing interventions for these clients *except*
   A. developing coping strategies with the client and family (such as relaxation techniques, controlled coughing techniques, and appropriate administration of oxygen) to manage dyspnea.
   B. conservative treatment of mild hemoptysis on an outpatient basis.
   C. teaching that warm humidified air and avoidance of cigarette smoke can help decrease the discomfort caused by irritation in the bronchial mucosa.
   D. teaching Kegel exercises and creating a schedule to incorporate them into a daily regimen.

5. A 66-year-old man is undergoing a course of radiation therapy as treatment for his lung cancer. Which *best* describes appropriate nursing actions?
   A. Teaching the client how to apply a special skin sealant dressing and nystatin powder for any open skin lesions in the treated area.
   B. Regular assessment of pain levels.
   C. Advising the clients to wear loose fitting clothes, keep the skin in the treatment area dry, and to avoid lotions and creams.
   D. Encouraging the client to use a heating pad for the muscle pain in the treated area.

ANSWERS

1. *Answer:* A
Rationale: Both extensive SCLC and stage II NSCLC have a poor prognosis for survival. However, clients with SCLC will live about 13 months, and those with NSCLC will live beyond that. Neither group will have many survivors beyond 2 years.

2. *Answer:* D
Rationale: Neither surgery nor radiotherapy alone is effective first-line treatment for SCLC. It is a fast-growing, aggressive tumor that is assumed to be systemic at the time of the diagnosis. Chemotherapy alone or with radiation therapy is therefore the standard treatment.

3. *Answer:* C
Rationale: More than 80% of lung cancers are associated with smoking; asbestos exposure is associated with roughly 3% to 4% of all lung cancers. Although the number of cases is small, lung cancer has been associated with radon gas exposure in smokers. There is no evidence that TB is linked to lung cancer.

4. *Answer:* D
Rationale: All statements but D are true. Kegel exercises help improve urinary inconti-

nence, which is generally not a problem associated with lung cancer.

5. *Answer:* C
Rationale: Pain is not a major side effect of radiation therapy. Standard guidelines for skin care during radiation therapy caution *against* using powders or any type of adhesive on the skin. Choice C describes the other standard skin care recommendations to be followed during radiation therapy.

BIBLIOGRAPHY

Brogden, J.M., & Nevidjon, B. (1995). Vinorelbine tartrate (Navelbine): Drug profile and nursing implications of a new vinca alkaloid. *Oncol Nurs Forum* 22(4), 635–646.

Bunn, P.A., & Kelly, K. (1995). New treatment agents for advanced small cell and non-small cell cancer. *Semin Oncol* 22(3), 53–63.

Glover, J., & Miaskowski, C. (1994). Small cell lung cancer: Pathophysiologic mechanisms and nursing implications. *Oncol Nurs Forum, 21*(1), 87–95.

Kubota, K., Furuse, K., & Kawahara, M., et al. (1994). Role of radiotherapy in combined modality treatment of locally advanced non-small cell lung cancer. *J Clin Oncol* 12(8), 1547–1552.

25

Nursing Care of the Client with Cancer of the Gastrointestinal Tract

Roberta Anne Strohl

Select the best answer for each of the following questions:

1. The most common side effect in patients receiving radiation therapy for colorectal cancer is
   A. nausea.
   B. diarrhea.
   C. bone marrow depression.
   D. intestinal obstruction.

2. Which tumor marker has been useful in monitoring for recurrence of colorectal cancer?
   A. AFP.
   B. HCG.
   C. CEA.
   D. OAF.

3. In which region does obstruction of the bowel occur most commonly in colon cancer?
   A. Sigmoid.
   B. Ascending.
   C. Transverse.
   D. Descending.

4. Increased risk of gastric cancer is associated with all of the following dietary factors *except*
   A. high fat and protein.
   B. salted meat and fish.
   C. low vitamin A and C.
   D. smoked foods.

5. The most common presenting symptom of esophageal cancer is
   A. cough.
   B. hematemesis.
   C. dysphagia.
   D. fatigue.

6. Persons with esophageal cancer are at risk for the development of second primary tumors of the head and neck area related to
   A. poor nutrition.
   B. side effects of therapy.
   C. common risk factors of tobacco and alcohol abuse.
   D. prior surgery.

ANSWERS

1. *Answer:* B
   Rationale: The rapid mitotic rate of gastrointestinal mucosa cells results in sensitivity to radiation.

2. *Answer:* C
   Rationale: Carcinoembryonic antigen (CEA) is generally elevated in persons with colon cancer. It is used to monitor the efficacy of treatment.

3. *Answer:* A
   Rationale: The obstruction is usually the result of the type of tumors characteristic of this area, which decrease the size of the bowel lumen.

4. *Answer:* A
   Rationale: Gastric cancer is not associated with low-fat and protein diets.

5. *Answer:* C
   Rationale: Dysphagia, the sensation of "food sticking," is the most common presentation of esophageal cancer.

6. *Answer:* C
   Rationale: Common risk factors for head and neck and esophageal cancers include alcohol and tobacco abuse.

BIBLIOGRAPHY

Boarini, J. (1990). Gastrointestinal cancer: Colon, rectum, and anus. In S.L. Groenwald, M.H. Frogge, M. Goodman, & C.H. Yarbro (eds.). *Cancer Nursing: Principles and Practice* (2nd ed.). Boston: Jones & Bartlett, pp. 792–805.

Holyoke, E.D. (1988). The role of the carcinoembryonic antigen in the management of colorectal cancer. In V.T. DeVita, S. Hellman, & S.A. Rosenberg (eds.). *Cancer: Principles and Practice of Oncology* (4th ed.). Philadelphia: JB Lippincott.

Pract Oncol Update 2(3), 1–11.

Messner, R.L., Gardner, S.S., & Webb, D.D. (1986). Early detection—the priority in colorectal cancer. *Cancer Nurs 9*(1), 8–14.

Roth, J., Lichter, A., Putnam, ••, Forastiere, A. (1993). Cancer of the esophagus. In V.T. DeVita, S. Hellman, & S.A. Rosenberg (eds.). *Cancer: Principles and Practice of Oncology* (4th ed.). Philadelphia: JB Lippincott, pp. 776–818.

Shank, B., Cohen, A.M., & Kelsen, D. (1989). Cancer of the anal region. In V.T. DeVita, S. Hellman, & S.A. Rosenberg (eds.). *Cancer: Principles and Practice of Oncology* (3rd ed.). Philadelphia: JB Lippincott, pp. 965–978.

26

Nursing Care of the Client with Leukemia

Molly J. Moran and Susan A. Ezzone

Select the best answer for each of the following questions:

1. All-*trans* retinoic acid is being used as initial treatment for
   A. acute myelocytic leukemia.
   B. acute promyelocytic leukemia.
   C. chronic myelogenous leukemia.
   D. acute myelomonocytic leukemia.

2. A positive Philadelphia chromosome is most commonly associated with
   A. acute myelocytic leukemia.
   B. hairy cell leukemia.
   C. chronic myelogenous leukemia.
   D. acute lymphocytic leukemia.

3. The central nervous system and testes are common sanctuary sites for which type of leukemia?
   A. Acute lymphocytic leukemia.
   B. Chronic lymphocytic leukemia.
   C. Hairy cell leukemia.
   D. Acute myelocytic leukemia.

4. Risk factors for leukemia include all of the following *except*
   A. exposure to severe temperature changes.
   B. previous treatment with an alkylating agent.
   C. exposure to radiation.
   D. exposure to specific viruses.

5. Induction treatment for AML usually consists of
   A. one single antineoplastic agent that is sensitive.
   B. a plant alkaloid agent with prednisone.
   C. diet therapy.
   D. cytarabine plus an anthracycline.

6. A 40-year-old woman was referred to a hematologist with a tentative diagnosis of AML. The client's only complaint was fatigue. Which of the following diagnostic tests would the hematologist most likely order first?
   A. Liver function tests.
   B. Uric acid.
   C. Lumbar puncture.
   D. Bone marrow aspirate and biopsy with special stains and immunophenotyping.

ANSWERS

1. *Answer:* B

Rationale: All-*trans* retinoic acid is used for treatment of promyelocytic leukemia to enhance differentiation rather than cause cytotoxicity. The other three types of leukemia mentioned in this question are treated initially with cytotoxic drugs.

2. *Answer:* C

Rationale: Approximately 95% of clients with CML are Philadelphia chromosome positive. This represents a translocation of the long arms of chromosomes 9 and 22. Clients who are Philadelphia chromosome positive usually have a better response to treatment and a longer survival rate than Philadelphia chromosome-negative clients.

3. *Answer:* A

Rationale: Lymphoblasts have a tendency to hide in the central nervous system and the testes. Even after remission has been obtained, leukemia cells can be found in these sites. Therefore the CNS is treated to prevent relapse of the disease at this site.

4. *Answer:* A

Rationale: Although the cause of leukemia is not known, factors that seem to have some relationship to the development of the disease include genetic factors, exposure to radiation, chemicals, drugs including alkylating agents, and viruses.

5. *Answer:* D

Rationale: Cytarabine, which is cell cycle specific, is used with an anthracycline, which is not cell cycle specific. The thought is that the anthracycline will entice the proliferating cells to enter the cell cycles.

6. *Answer:* D

Rationale: Uric acid and lactic dehydrogenase levels may be elevated. A bone marrow biopsy and aspirate with special stains is done. These tests show the cellularity of the marrow and will denote the presence of Auer rods, which are diagnostic of AML. Special stains such as Sudan Black and peroxidase are used to diagnose AML. The presence of leukemic cells in the CNS is more common in ALL rather than AML.

BIBLIOGRAPHY

Deisseroth, A.B., Andreeff, M., Champlin, R., et al. (1993). Chronic leukemias. In V.T. DeVita, Jr., S. Hellman, & S.A. Rosenberg (eds.). *Cancer: Principles and Practice of Oncology* (4th ed.). Philadelphia: JB Lippincott, pp. 1965–1980.

Forman, S.J., Blume, K.G., & Thomas, E.D. (1994). *Bone Marrow Transplantation.* Boston: Blackwell Scientific Publications.

Groenwald, S.L., Frogge, M.H., Goodman, M., & Yarbro, C.G. (eds.). (1990). Leukemia. In *Comprehensive Cancer Nursing Review* (2nd ed.). Boston: Jones & Bartlett, pp. 448–464.

Haeuber, D., & Spross, J. (1994). Protective mechanisms: Bone marrow. In B.L. Johnson & J. Gross (eds.). *Handbook of Oncology Nursing* (2nd ed.). Boston: Jones & Bartlett, pp. 373–380.

Keating, M.J., Estey, E., & Kantarijian, H. (1993). Acute leukemia. In V.T. DeVita, Jr., S. Hellman, & S.A. Rosenberg (eds.). *Cancer: Principles and Practice of Oncology* (4th ed.). Philadelphia: JB Lippincott, pp. 1938–1959.

Wujcik, D., Viele, C.S., & Caudell, K.A. (1996). Leukemia management strategies: The next generation. *Oncol Nurs Forum 23*(3), 477–502.

Yeager, K.A., & Miaskowski, C. (1994). Advances in understanding the mechanisms and management of acute myelogenous leukemia. *Oncol Nurs Forum 21*(3), 541–548.

27

Nursing Care of the Client with Lymphoma and Multiple Myeloma

Joyce Alexander

Select the best answer for each of the following questions:

1. Mr. J. presents at his physician's office with enlarged lymph nodes and a history of night sweats. Although the physician suspects Hodgkin's disease, which of the following will be *required* to make a diagnosis of Hodgkin's disease?
   A. Fevers accompanying night sweats.
   B. A history of infections within 3 months of presentation with enlarged nodes.
   C. An excisional biopsy with Reed-Sternberg cells noted by the pathologist.
   D. A chest x-ray film, CT scans of the chest and abdomen, and lymphogram.

2. Pain in a client with multiple myeloma commonly results from
   A. intestinal obstruction due to enlarging soft tissue mass.
   B. neural infiltration of plasma cells.
   C. lytic bone lesions.
   D. marrow infiltration.

3. Mr. J. is determined to have stage III B Hodgkin's disease. The next step in his treatment is likely to be
   A. combination chemotherapy with MOPP (mechlorethamine, vincristine, procarbazine, and prednisone) or ABVD (doxorubicin, bleomycin, vinblastine, dacarbazine).
   B. wait and observe the lymph nodes to see if continued growth occurs.

   C. concurrent radiation and chemotherapy with ABF (doxorubicin, bleomycin, and fluorouracil).
   D. radiation therapy alone.

4. Mr. Y. is admitted to the hospital for his first dose of combination chemotherapy for lymphoma. He states, "The doctor said most of my treatments would be given in the clinic. Why must I be in the hospital this time?" What is your best response?
   A. "Because lymphoma responds so well to chemotherapy the dying lymphoma cells sometimes cause problems with the first treatment. We like to watch for and prevent problems."
   B. "Sometimes people have a lot of nausea with these treatments and we have to give you lots of medicine, especially with the first treatment."
   C. "It is important to monitor for allergic reactions with the first treatment. You may need medications for an allergic reaction."
   D. "Everyone comes to the hospital for their first treatment on these drugs. I guess it is because your white blood cell counts drop immediately and you may get an infection and require antibiotics."

5. Mr. S., a 17-year-old male client, is scheduled to receive initial chemotherapy for Hodgkin's disease. After watching a video on chemo-

152

therapy, he makes the following comment to his nurse, "I guess taking chemotherapy means I will never have children." Which of the following is the most appropriate nursing intervention?

    A. The nurse states, "I wouldn't worry about it" and starts Mr. S.'s chemotherapy.

    B. The nurse tells the client that some people have problems but that he may not and offers to call the doctor to talk with him further if the client wishes. When the client does not make further comment, the nurse proceeds with chemotherapy.

    C. The nurse discusses sperm banking, provides the client with information, notifies the physician that the client has concerns, and delays the chemotherapy until the client can make a decision.

    D. The nurse documents in her notes that the client has concerns and may need a consultation for sperm banking after this admission and then proceeds with chemotherapy.

6. Mr. R. has a diagnosis of multiple myeloma and has been receiving oral melphalan and pred-nisone over a period of several months. The nurse notes a weight loss of 10 pounds in the past month. The client states, "The doctor said my blood protein was high so I was trying to avoid protein in my diet." The best nursing intervention is to

    A. tell the client that he is doing very well to avoid protein since his blood protein was high and congratulate him on his weight loss.

    B. explain to the client that the high blood protein is not a problem but that he should continue his diet as before except for adding more fat. Consult the dietitian for a high-fat diet to help the client regain lost weight.

    C. explain to the client that the protein in his blood is from the myeloma, not his diet, and that he needs a well-balanced diet. Consult the dietitian to help the client increase his caloric intake with an adequate protein intake and a balanced diet.

    D. give the client a pamphlet on the importance of nutrition for cancer clients and ask him to call if he has questions.

NOTES

ANSWERS

1. *Answer:* C

Rationale: The presence of Reed-Sternberg cells on biopsy is required to make a diagnosis of Hodgkin's disease. Fevers accompanying night sweats and frequent infections before diagnosis may be symptomatic of Hodgkin's disease but are not diagnostic. The chest radiograph, CT scans, and lymphogram may be required for staging but not for diagnosis.

2. *Answer:* C

Rationale: Lytic bone lesions are the most common cause of pain in multiple myeloma. Although the marrow may be involved, this is not a common cause of pain. Neural infiltration and intestinal obstruction are not common in multiple myeloma.

3. *Answer:* A

Rationale: For stage III B Hodgkin's disease appropriate treatment is combination chemotherapy with MOPP or ABVD. Concurrent radiation and chemotherapy is generally reserved for stage II with bulky mediastinal disease and would not use the regimen listed in any case. Radiation alone is reserved for stage I or II without bulky mediastinal disease.

4. *Answer:* A

Rationale: Tumor lysis syndrome is common with the first treatment of lymphoma. Allergic reactions are not common; neutropenia occurs several days later; and nausea is no more a problem than with other chemotherapy.

5. *Answer:* C

Rationale: The client has raised an issue for which the nurse should provide more information. He will likely need some private time to make a decision or to call significant others for help with the decision. Sperm banking should be done before the first chemotherapy session if at all possible.

6. *Answer:* C

Rationale: The physician was referring to the myeloma (M) protein levels in the client's blood. The client needs a nutritious, well-balanced diet and should not be encouraged to lose weight during chemotherapy treatment. The nurse should clarify the misconception and then provide referral or information on a nutritious diet. Giving the client a pamphlet without clarifying issues would not be helpful.

BIBLIOGRAPHY

Alexander, J. (1998). Nursing care of the client with lymphoma and multiple myeloma. In J.K. Itano & K.N. Taoka (eds.). *Core Curriculum for Oncology Nursing* (3rd ed.). Philadelphia: WB Saunders, pp. 496–503.

Clark, J. (1994). Multiple myeloma. In S. Otto (ed.). *Oncology Nursing* (2nd ed.). St. Louis: Mosby, pp. 356–360.

Longo, D., DeVita, V., Jaffe, E., Mauch, P., & Urba, W. (1993). Lymphocytic lymphomas. In V. DeVita, S. Hellman, & S. Rosenberg (eds.). *Cancer: Principles and Practice of Oncology* (4th ed.). Philadelphia: JB Lippincott, pp. 1859–1916.

Sheridan, C. (1996). Multiple myeloma. *Semin Oncol Nurs 12*(1), 59–69.

28

Nursing Care of the Client with Bone and Soft Tissue Cancers

Ellen Carr

Select the best answer for each of the following questions:

1. Treatment goals for bone cancer include all of the following *except*
   A. preserving functioning.
   B. recalcification.
   C. avoiding amputation.
   D. removing the entire tumor from the body.

2. An early sign or symptom of a soft tissue tumor is
   A. pain.
   B. fatigue.
   C. swelling.
   D. discolored skin.

3. Soft tissue sarcomas frequently spread first to the
   A. lung.
   B. brain.
   C. stomach.
   D. kidney.

4. When there is a suspicion of osteosarcoma, a laboratory finding that leads to the diagnosis is
   A. elevated WBC.
   B. elevated serum alkaline phosphatase.
   C. hypercalcemia.
   D. low creatinine.

5. Rehabilitation from soft tissue or bone tumor treatment usually includes all of the following *except*
   A. management of phantom limb pain.
   B. coordination of fine motor movement.
   C. strengthening of muscle tone.
   D. energy conservation.

ANSWERS

1. *Answer:* B

   Rationale: Recalcification of the tissue is not a treatment goal. Treatment goals include A, C, and D. As a treatment goal, recalcification does not stop or slow the growth of bone cancer. Recalcification may not be timely, precise, or thorough enough to treat the tumor or its growth.

2. *Answer:* C

   Rationale: Swelling is the cardinal sign of a soft tissue tumor. Pain, fatigue, and discolored skin occur later in soft tissue tumor growth.

3. *Answer:* A

   Rationale: The lung is the most frequent site of initial soft tissue tumor migration. Soft tissue spread can be distant from the site of origin, but the most common initial spread is to the lung.

4. *Answer:* B

   Rationale: Elevated serum alkaline phosphatase indicates increased osteoblastic activity, an indication of tumor growth. The other laboratory findings do not indicate increased osteoblastic activity. Osteoblastic activity indicates osteosarcoma tumor growth.

5. *Answer:* B

   Rationale: Gross motor movements are more likely to be the focus of rehabilitation plans. Choices A, C, and D are part of rehabilitation after soft tissue or bone tumor treatment.

BIBLIOGRAPHY

Chang, S. (1994). Bone cancers and soft tissue sarcomas. In S. Otto (ed.). *Oncology Nursing.* St. Louis: Mosby, p. 59.

Dorfman, H., & Czerniak, B. (1995). Bone cancers. *Cancer 75*(1 suppl), 203.

Malawer, M., Link., M., & Donaldson, S. (1993). Sarcomas of bone. In V. Devita, Jr., S. Hellman, & S. Rosenberg (eds.). *Cancer: Principles and Practice of Oncology* (4th ed.). Philadelphia: JB Lippincott, p. 1509.

Paisecki, P. (1993). Bone and soft tissue sarcoma. In S.L. Groenwald, M.H. Frogge, M. Goodman, & C.H. Yarbro (eds.). *Cancer Nursing Principles and Practice* (3rd ed.). Boston: Jones & Bartlett, p. 877.

Renard, J., Veth, R., & Pruszczynksi, M. (1995). Ewing's sarcoma of bone: oncologic and functional results. *J Surg Oncol 60*(4), 250.

Zalupski, M., & Baker, L. (1995). Systemic adjuvant chemotherapy for soft tissue sarcomas. *Hematol Oncol Clin North Am 9*(4), 787.

NOTES

29

Nursing Care of the Client with HIV-Related Cancer

Patricia F. Jassak

Select the best answer for each of the following questions:

1. AIDS-related Kaposi's sarcoma (KS) differs from classic KS in that
   A. classic KS is generally seen only in the pediatric population.
   B. there is no characteristic pattern of presentation seen in AIDS-related KS.
   C. lesions associated with classic KS are less than 2 cm in diameter.
   D. women do not develop AIDS-related KS.

2. Symptoms associated with primary central nervous system (CNS) AIDS-related lymphoma include all of the following *except*
   A. altered mental status.
   B. seizure disorders.
   C. hemiparesis.
   D. oliguria.

3. All of the following are considered appropriate treatment interventions for AIDS-related lymphoma *except*
   A. surgery.
   B. chemotherapy.
   C. radiotherapy.
   D. biologic response modifiers.

4. Most AIDS-related lymphomas are
   A. T-cell, low-grade.
   B. B-cell, high-grade.
   C. T-cell, high-grade.
   D. B-cell, low-grade.

ANSWERS

1. *Answer:* B
   Rationale: Classic KS is generally seen on the lower extremities, usually distal to the knee, typically in elderly men. HIV-related KS can present in virtually any organ system.

2. *Answer:* D
   Rationale: Oliguria is not caused by a CNS deficit.

3. *Answer:* A
   Rationale: Surgical treatment is contraindicated in the typical presence of disseminated disease associated with AIDS-related lymphoma.

4. *Answer:* B
   Rationale: Most clients who present with HIV-related lymphoma have B-cell tumors of high-grade histologic type because of the lack of effective T-cell mediated immune regulation.

BIBLIOGRAPHY

Doll, D.C., & Ringenberg, Q.S. (1989). Lymphomas associated with HIV infection. *Semin Oncol Nurs 5*(4), 255–262.

Grady, C. (1988). Host defense mechanisms: An overview. *Semin Oncol Nurs 4*(2) 86–94.

Halloran, J. (1994). HIV-related malignancies. In D. Grimes & D. Grimes (eds.). *HIV/AIDS Nursing Care.* St. Louis: Mosby–Year Book, pp. 140–152.

Halloran, J.P., & Hughes, A.M. (1991). Knowledge deficit related to prevention and early detection of HIV disease. In J.C. McNally, E.T. Somerville, C. Miaskowski, & M. Rostad (eds.). *Guidelines for Oncology Nursing Practice* (2nd ed.). Philadelphia: WB Saunders, pp. 47–54.

Kaplan, L.D., & Northfelt, D.W. (1997). Malignancies associated with AIDS. In M.A. Sande & P.A. Volberding (eds.). *The Medical Management of AIDS.* Philadelphia: WB Saunders, pp. 413–439.

Lovejoy, N.C. (1988). The pathophysiology of AIDS. *Oncol Nurs Forum 15*(5), 563–571.

McMahon, K.M., & Coyne, N. (1989). Symptom management in patients with AIDS. *Semin Oncol Nurs 5*(4), 289–301.

Selik, R.M., Chu, S.Y., & Ward, J.W. (1995). Trends in infections and cancers among persons dying of HIV infection in the U.S. from 1987–1992. *Ann Intern Med 123*, 933–936.

Ungvarski, P.J., & Flaskerud, J.H. (eds.). (1999). *HIV/AIDS: A Guide to Primary Care Management* (4th ed.). Philadelphia: WB Saunders.

NOTES

30

Nursing Care of the Client with Genital Cancer

Lana Hlava Renaud

Select the best answer for each of the following questions:

1. The *most common* presenting symptom of endometrial cancer is
   A. acute abdominal pain.
   B. increased abdominal girth.
   C. abnormal vaginal bleeding.
   D. milky vaginal drainage.

2. A client is receiving paclitaxel and cisplatin for ovarian cancer. In developing her care plan, you would include assessment of all of the following side effects *except*
   A. alopecia.
   B. stomatitis.
   C. nausea and vomiting.
   D. neuropathies.

3. You are caring for a woman with recently diagnosed endometrial cancer. She tells you she does not understand how she can have cancer when her Papanicolaou (Pap) smear was negative 8 months ago. Which of the following responses is the most appropriate?
   A. Many Pap smears are not interpreted correctly.
   B. Endometrial cancer may develop in a short time.
   C. The Pap specimen may have been obtained incorrectly.
   D. Pap smears do not commonly detect endometrial cancer.

4. Personal risk factors for endometrial cancer include all of the following *except*
   A. obesity.
   B. diabetes.
   C. estrogen replacement without progestational agents.
   D. hypotension.

5. The wife of a client with testicular cancer stops you in the hall. Her husband is receiving his first cycle of chemotherapy. She tells you she doesn't know what she'll do when he dies. In forming your response, you remember that the prognosis for testicular cancer is
   A. highly variable depending on stage.
   B. highly variable depending on histology.
   C. excellent and considered a curable disease.
   D. less than a 70% survival rate.

6. All of the following are appropriate screening procedures for reproductive cancers *except*
   A. monthly testicular self-examinations.
   B. initial Pap smear with bimanual pelvic examination at age 18 years or on initiation of sexual intercourse.
   C. endometrial aspiration or biopsy.
   D. serial CA-125 levels for all women age 18 and older.

ANSWERS

1. *Answer:* C
   Rationale: Abdominal discomfort and increasing girth are significant symptoms of ovarian cancer. Milky vaginal drainage may occur with cervical cancer. Twenty percent of postmenopausal bleeding is related to endometrial cancer.

2. *Answer:* B
   Rationale: Cisplatin and paclitaxel are two commonly used drugs in the management of ovarian cancer. Both drugs have a low potential for causing stomatitis.

3. *Answer:* D
   Rationale: Exfoliated malignant cells from the endometrium are rarely detected on a cervical sampling (the Pap test). A Pap smear is a screening test for cervical intraepithelial neoplasias or invasive cervical cancer.

4. *Answer:* D
   Rationale: Hypertension is a personal risk factor.

5. *Answer:* C
   Rationale: Testicular cancer is a model for a curable solid tumor.

6. *Answer:* D
   Rationale: Screening CA-l25 determinations in women supplemented by transvaginal ultrasound remains controversial but is sometimes used in high-risk women.

BIBLIOGRAPHY

Berek, J.S., & Hacker, N.F. (1994). *Practical Gynecologic Oncology* (2nd ed.). Baltimore: Williams & Wilkins.

Broadwell, D.C., & Jackson, B.S. (eds.). (1982). *Principles of Ostomy Care.* St. Louis: CV Mosby.

DeVita, V.T., Jr., Hellman, S., & Rosenberg, S.A. (eds.). (1993). *Cancer: Principles and Practice of Oncology* (4th ed.). Philadelphia: JB Lippincott.

DiSaia, P.J., & Creasman, W.T. (1993). *Clinical Gynecologic Oncology* (4th ed.). St. Louis: Mosby–Year Book.

Hawkins, C., & Miaskowski, C. (1996). Testicular cancer: A review. *Oncol Nurs Forum 23,* 1203–1211.

Ibbotson, T., & Wyke, S. (1995). A review of cervical cancer and cervical screening: Implications for nursing practice. *J Adv Nurs 22,* 745–752.

Lovejoy, N.C. (1994). Precancerous and cancerous cervical lesions: The multicultural "male" risk factor. *Oncol Nurs Forum 21,* 497–504.

McCorkle, R., Grant, M., Frank-Stromberg, M., & Baird, S. (eds.). (1996). *Cancer Nursing: A Comprehensive Textbook* (2nd ed.). Philadelphia: WB Saunders.

NIH Consensus Development Panel on Ovarian Cancer. (1995). Ovarian cancer: Screening, treatment, and follow-up. *JAMA 273*(6) 491–497.

Ozols, R. (1995). Current status of chemotherapy for ovarian cancer. *Semin Oncol 22*(5 suppl 2), 61–66.

Rubin, P. (ed.). (1993). *Clincal Oncology: A Multidisciplinary Approach for Physicians and Students* (7th ed.). Philadelphia: WB Saunders.

Wright, T.C., Jr., & Richart, R.M. (1992). Pathogenesis and diagnosis of preinvasive lesion of the lower genital tract. In W.J. Hoskins, C.A. Perez, & R.C. Young (eds.). *Principles and Practice of Gynecologic Oncology.* Philadelphia: JB Lippincott, pp. 509–536.

Zacharias, D.R., Gilg, C.A., & Foxall, M.J. (1994). Quality of life and coping in patients with gynecologic cancer and their spouses. *Oncol Nurs Forum 21,* 1699–1706.

31

Nursing Care of the Client with Skin Cancer

Alice J. Longman

Select the best answer for each of the following questions:

1. In the initial treatment of skin cancer, which of the standard therapies for the treatment of cancer is most effective?
   - A. Surgical excision.
   - B. Radiation therapy.
   - C. Chemotherapy.
   - D. Hormonal therapy/biotherapy.

2. Which of the following lesion types has the highest risk of recurrence?
   - A. Basal cell carcinoma.
   - B. Squamous cell carcinoma.
   - C. Nodular melanoma.
   - D. Superficial spreading melanoma.

3. In counseling clients and families about continued care after treatment for skin cancer, which of the following activities is the *most* important?
   - A. Monitoring site where the lesion occurred.
   - B. Monthly self-examination of the skin.
   - C. Updating family history of skin cancers.
   - D. Collecting information about skin cancer from national cancer-related organizations.

4. In teaching about the prevention of skin cancer, the *major areas* to be included initially are
   - A. length of exposure to sunlight, use of sunscreen (sun protection factor [SPF] of 15 or more), use of protective clothing, and use of sunglasses.
   - B. time of day during sun exposure, time of year of sun exposure, weather conditions during sun exposure, and recreational activities.
   - C. skin type, genetic history, family pedigree about skin cancer, and use of tanning parlors.
   - D. skin assessment, effect of altitude during sun exposure, time of year during sun exposure, and time of day of sun exposure.

ANSWERS

1. *Answer:* A

Rationale: Although all of the standard therapies may be used during the course of treatment for skin cancer, particularly malignant melanoma, surgical excision is used 90% of the time. In the treatment of malignant melanoma, it may be necessary to remove nearby lymph nodes, although this is controversial.

2. *Answer:* C

Rationale: Equally high cure rates with either surgery or radiation can be achieved for basal cell carcinoma and squamous cell carcinoma. Although a possibility of recurrence exists with either one, continued surveillance improves the ability to detect it readily. The most important prognostic feature in malignant melanoma is the size of the lesion at the time of diagnosis. Nodular melanoma has the highest risk of recurrence and metastasis.

3. *Answer:* B

Rationale: Evaluation at regular intervals by a physician or nurse is important for those who have received treatment for skin cancer. Clients and families are instructed to assume responsibility for their own care. One of the most important activities is to do systematic, monthly skin self-examination.

4. *Answer:* A

Rationale: Exposure to sunlight should be limited between 10 AM and 3 PM in high-intensity sun areas. Sunscreens (SPF of 15 or more) are recommended with frequent reapplications during prolonged sun exposure. Protective clothing and sunglasses are also recommended during prolonged exposure to sunlight. All of these are important in teaching about the prevention of skin cancer.

BIBLIOGRAPHY

Friedman, R.J., Rigel, D.S., Silverman, M.K., Kopf, A.W., & Vossaert, K.A. (1991). Malignant melanoma in the 1990s: The continued importance of early detection and the role of physician examination and self-examination of the skin. *CA Cancer J Clin 41*, 201–226.

Ketcham, A.S., & Balch, C.M. (1985). Classification and staging systems. In C.M. Balch, G.W. Milton, H.M. Shaw, & S.J. Soong (eds.). *Cutaneous Melanoma.* Philadelphia: JB Lippincott, pp. 52–62.

Loescher, L.J. (1993). Skin cancer prevention and screening update. *Semin Oncol Nurs 8*, 184–187.

Longman, A.J. (1996). Malignant melanoma. In M.C. Liebman & D. Camp-Sorrell (eds.). *Multimodal Therapy in Oncology Nursing.* St. Louis: Mosby–Year Book, pp. 271–280.

Longman, A.J. (1996). Skin cancers. In R. McCorkle, M. Grant, M. Frank-Stromborg, & S.B. Baird (eds). *Cancer Nursing: A Comprehensive Textbook* (2nd ed.). Philadelpha: WB Saunders, pp. 860–869.

Longman, A.J. (1998). Nursing care of the client with skin cancer. In J. Itano & K. Taoka (eds.). *Core Curriculum for Oncology Nursing* (3rd ed.). Philadelphia: WB Saunders, pp. 552–560.

Vargo, N.L. (1991). Basal and squamous cell carcinoma: An overview. *Semin Oncol Nurs 7*, 13–25.

32

Nursing Care of the Client with Cancer of the Neurologic System

Marva Bohen

Select the best answer for each of the following questions:

1. Which of the following is *not* a common presenting symptom for clients with a brain tumor?
   A. Seizure.
   B. Unilateral headache.
   C. Fever.
   D. Hemiparesis.

2. Which of the following statements is true regarding high grade astrocytomas?
   A. They metastasize frequently to the liver or lungs or both.
   B. They infiltrate into surrounding brain tissue.
   C. They are usually encapsulated.
   D. They respond well to standard chemotherapy.

3. The most common type of malignant brain tumors arises from
   A. neurons.
   B. astrocytes.
   C. oligodendrocytes.
   D. lymphatic tissues in the brain.

4. A client presents with a history of lung cancer and new onset of radicular pain of the left leg and spinal tenderness in the lower back. What nursing assessments are critical for this client?
   A. Pupil checks.
   B. Function of bowel and bladder.
   C. Cranial nerve examination.
   D. Upper extremity strength.

ANSWERS

1. *Answer:* C
Rationale: Seizure is the most common presenting symptom. Headaches and unilateral hemiparesis are also fairly common. Fever is not a common presenting symptom.

2. *Answer:* B
Rationale: High-grade astrocytomas infiltrate surrounding brain tissue and usually are not encapsulated. They rarely metastasize outside the central nervous system. Most chemotherapy agents given intravenously or orally do not cross the blood-brain barrier.

3. *Answer:* B
Rationale: Almost half of all malignant brain tumors arise from astrocytes. Malignant tumors arising from neurons are rare. Oligodendrogliomas account for only about 5% of malignant tumors. There are no lymphatic tissues in the brain.

4. *Answer:* B
Rationale: Dysfunctions of bladder and bowel and deterioration of lower extremity motor and sensory function would indicate spinal cord compression and require emergency intervention. The other nursing measures would not assess this potential problem.

BIBLIOGRAPHY

Bohen, M. (1997). Neurological cancer. In J.K Itano & K.N. Taoka (eds.). *Core Curriculum for Oncology Nursing* (3rd ed.). Philadelphia: WB Saunders, pp. 561–578.
McCorkle, R., Grant, M., Frank-Stromborg, M., & Baird, S. (eds.). (1996). *Cancer Nursing: A Comprehensive Textbook* (2nd ed.). Philadelphia: WB Saunders.
Segal, G. (1996). *A Primer of Brain Tumors* (6th ed.). Chicago: American Brain Tumor Association.
Wen, P.Y., & Black, P.M. (eds.). (1995). Brain tumors in adults [entire issue]. *Neurol Clin 13*(4).

NOTES

33

Nursing Care of the Client with Head and Neck Cancer

Ryan R. Iwamoto

Select the best answer for each of the following questions:

1. Risk factors for head and neck cancer include all of the following *except*
   A. smoking.
   B. alcohol consumption.
   C. high-fat diet.
   D. Epstein-Barr virus.

2. A client is surgically treated for a T3, N1, M0 cancer of the true vocal cord. The resulting dysfunction includes all of the following *except*
   A. aphonia.
   B. permanent tracheal stoma.
   C. inability to blow out candles on a birthday cake.
   D. raspy voice.

3. A client returns for the first office visit after a right composite neck resection with complaints of right shoulder pain and limited range of motion (90 degrees). An appropriate nursing action is to
   A. obtain a shoulder x-ray for a suspected lytic lesion in the shoulder.
   B. immobilize the arm and shoulder in a sling.
   C. obtain a physical therapy consultation for shoulder exercises.
   D. give the client a steroid injection in the shoulder.

4. Oral care after head and neck surgery would include
   A. rinsing the oral cavity with half-and-half peroxide and normal saline solution.
   B. cleansing the oral cavity with lemon glycerine swabs.
   C. brushing the teeth with a hard-bristled toothbrush.
   D. suctioning the oral cavity with high-pressure vacuum catheters.

ANSWERS

1. *Answer:* C

Rationale: Smoking and alcohol consumption are the classic risk factors for cancers of the oral cavity, oropharynx, and larynx. The Epstein-Barr virus is associated with cancers of the nasopharynx. A high-fat diet has not been identified as a risk factor for head and neck cancers.

2. *Answer:* D

Rationale: Surgical treatment of a T3, N1, M0 cancer of the true vocal cord requires a total laryngectomy. Resulting dysfunction includes loss of voice (aphonia), permanent tracheal stoma, and no air source from the lungs to the mouth. Therefore the client would be unable to blow out candles on a birthday cake. A supraglottic laryngectomy would result in a raspy voice and initially some degree of aspiration.

3. *Answer:* C

Rationale: A composite resection includes a neck dissection with resultant shoulder droop and forward curvature of the spine. Physical therapy for range of motion and resistive exercises are the best initial treatment to restore function and decrease pain. It is highly unlikely that the client has a lytic lesion of the shoulder. Immobilization of the arm and shoulder will exacerbate the client's shoulder problems. Because this condition is a result of the resection of the spinal accessory nerve and the sternocleidomastoid muscles rather than inflammatory changes, steroid injections would be of minimal benefit.

4. *Answer:* A

Rationale: Oral care after head and neck surgery includes gentle cleansing with gravity gavage or jet-spray dental cleansing system, using toothettes to remove mucus crusts, and rinsing with half-and-half peroxide and normal saline solution. Lemon glycerine swabs can cause mucosal drying because of the glycerine and should therefore be avoided. Hard-bristled toothbrushes and suctioning with high-pressure vacuum catheters can injure the mucosa and should be avoided.

BIBLIOGRAPHY

Baker, C.A. (1992). Factors associated with rehabilitation in head and neck cancer. *Cancer Nursing 15*(6), 395–400.

Iwamoto, R.R. (1997). Nursing care of the client with head and neck cancer. In J.K. Itano & K.N. Taoka (eds.). *Core Curriculum for Oncology Nursing* (3rd ed.). Philadelphia: WB Saunders, pp. 579–604.

Madeya, M.L. (1996). Oral complications from cancer therapy: Pathophysiology and secondary complications (part 1). *Oncol Nurs Forum 23*(5), 801–807.

Madeya, M.L. (1996). Oral complications from cancer therapy: Nursing implications for assessment and treatment (part 2). *Oncol Nurs Forum 23*(5), 808–819.

National Institutes of Health. (1989). Oral complications of cancer therapies: Diagnosis, prevention, and treatment. *Consensus Development Conference Statement 7*(7), 1–11.

Reese, J.L. (1996). Head and neck cancers. In R. McCorkle, M. Grant, M. Frank-Stromborg, & S.B. Baird (eds.). *Cancer Nursing: A Comprehensive Textbook* (2nd ed.). Philadelphia: WB Saunders, pp. 773–795.

Shah, J.P., & Lydiatt, W. (1995). Treatment of cancer of the head and neck. *CA Cancer J Clin 45*(6), 352–368.

Spitz, M.R. (1994). Epidemiology and risk factors for head and neck cancer. *Semin Oncol Nurs 21*(3), 281–288.

34

Nursing Implications of Surgical Treatment

Thomas J. Szopa

Select the best answer for each of the following questions:

1. An excisional biopsy means that the client
   A. had a portion of tissue removed at the tumor margin for examination.
   B. had an aspiration of fluid or tissue with a needle.
   C. had the complete removal of the tumor with little or no margin of surrounding normal tissue removed.
   D. had a large portion of her breast, which included the tumor, removed.

2. The definition of a wide excision or "en bloc" dissection is
   A. removal of a wedge of tissue from a larger tumor mass.
   B. obtaining a core of tissue through a needle.
   C. removal of tumor, any tissues containing primary nodal drainage area, and any involved contiguous structures.
   D. excision of the entire suspected lesion.

3. A 45-year-old client with a history of moderate ulcerative colitis for more than 12 years is scheduled for a total colectomy with ileostomy creation. The surgeon described this surgery as "prophylactic" cancer surgery, which is defined as
   A. the reconstruction of anatomic defects created by cancer surgery to improve function and cosmetic appearance.
   B. surgery performed on organs that have an extremely high risk of developing a subsequent cancer.

   C. the insertion of various therapeutic hardware during active treatment periods to facilitate the delivery of treatment and increase client comfort.
   D. the removal of hormonal influence of the cancer.

4. Radiation therapy before cancer surgery can
   A. improve tumor resectability and alter the extent of surgery needed.
   B. alter the extent of surgery needed but increase the functional disabilities after therapy.
   C. provide more appealing options to clients but decrease treatment outcomes.
   D. improve treatment outcomes but increase the functional disabilities after therapy.

5. A client was just visited by her surgeon. The nurse enters her room and finds her preoccupied and anxious. On questioning, she informs the nurse that her surgeon had recommended a simple lumpectomy and a course of radiation therapy versus a modified radical mastectomy. She continues by telling the nurse that she thought a mastectomy was the only way to treat breast cancer and requests an explanation. What would be the nurse's appropriate response?
   A. Clients have choices in primary treatment based on the stage and grade of their disease. The nurse explains that combination therapy reduces the amount of tissue to be removed while having the

same effect on the cancer. The nurse encourages her to speak further with her doctor.

B. Lumpectomy and radiation therapy are considered primary therapy, and mastectomy is a salvage therapy.

C. Lumpectomy is a cytoreductive therapy so that the primary therapy, radiation, would be more effective.

D. If her surgeon recommends a particular treatment, she would be wise to follow his recommendations.

NOTES

ANSWERS

1. *Answer:* C

Rationale: Excisional therapy is used on small, accessible tumors. The entire mass is removed with little or no margin of surrounding normal tissue. In some cases, excisional biopsy alone is definitive therapy. Other responses are incorrect definitions.

2. *Answer:* C

Rationale: Response A is an incisional therapy. Response B is a needle biopsy. Response D is an excisional biopsy.

3. *Answer:* B

Rationale: Surgical removal of a particular body tissue or organ is recommended if that tissue or organ has a high risk for the occurrence of cancer within it. A 10+-year history of chronic ulcerative colitis, along with the client's age, increases the risk significantly for colorectal cancer. Responses A, C, and D are definitions of other types of surgeries performed for cancer.

4. *Answer:* A

Rationale: Shrinkage of the tumor will occur whereby its margins will be more discernible by the surgeon and more easily removed. This reduces the impact on surrounding tissues. Responses B, C, and D are incorrect because the goal is optimum cancer treatment outcomes with minimal disability.

5. *Answer:* A

Rationale: The treatment principle is correct, and the nurse supports more discussion with the physician to help the client be more informed of the decision she makes. Responses B and C provide incorrect definitions of the role of these therapies in breast cancer treatment for this client. Response D does not support informed consent for this client or address her informational needs.

BIBLIOGRAPHY

Frogge, M.H. (1997). Surgical therapy. In S. Groenwald, M. Frogge, R. Goodman, & C. Yarbro (eds.). *Cancer Nursing: Principles and Practice* (4th ed.). Boston: Jones & Bartlett, pp. 229–246.

Markman, M. (1995). Surgery for support and palliation in patients with malignant disease. *Semin Oncol 22*(2 suppl 3), 91–94.

Polomono, R., Weintraub, F.N., & Wurster, A. (1994). Surgical critical care for cancer patients. *Semin Oncol Nurs 10*(3), 165–176.

Szopa, T.J. (1998). Nursing implications of surgical treatment. In J.K. Itano & K.N. Taoka (eds.). *Core Curriculum for Oncology Nursing* (3rd ed.). Philadelphia: WB Saunders, pp. 605–615.

Weintraub, F., & Neumark, D. (1996). Surgical oncology. In R. McCorkle, M. Grant, M. Frank-Stromborg, & S. Baird (eds.). *Cancer Nursing: A Comprehensive Textbook* (2nd ed.). Philadelphia: WB Saunders, pp. 315–330.

35

Nursing Implications of Radiation Therapy

Ellen Sitton

Select the best answer for each of the following questions:

1. Which of the following statements best describes the radiobiology of treatment with ionizing radiation?
   A. Ionizing radiation injures cellular DNA of both normal and cancer tissues.
   B. Only normal cells can repair damage to DNA.
   C. Altered DNA always produces hereditary changes.
   D. Cells that are lethally damaged by ionizing radiation die within an hour of the radiation dose.

2. Which of the following statements about radiosensitivity is *not true*?
   A. Radiosensitivity of a tissue is characteristic of the tissue regardless of whether the ionizing radiation is delivered as external beam radiation, sealed source radiation therapy, or unsealed source radiation therapy.
   B. Normal cells vary in their sensitivity to ionizing radiation, but all cancer cells have approximately the same degree of sensitivity to ionizing radiation.
   C. In general, well-oxygenated cells are more sensitive to ionizing radiation than hypoxic cells of the same type.

   D. Tissues that are considered late responding tissues generally do not demonstrate observable effects during the course of radiation therapy.

3. A 41-year-old premenopausal woman with cervical cancer is treated with 4500 cGy external beam treatment to the pelvis through anterior and posterior fields before intracavitary sealed source application. Which of the following side effects is least likely to be a result of external beam irradiation to the pelvis in this client?
   A. Fatigue.
   B. Cystitis symptoms.
   C. Menopausal symptoms.
   D. Nausea and vomiting.

4. A 69-year-old man with multiple bone metastases from prostate cancer has just received the radioactive isotope strontium 89 for relief of bone pain. The client is an inpatient. Which of the following radiation precautions would not be necessary on the first day for this client?
   A. Flush the toilet three times to dispose of urine.
   B. Consider all body fluids to be radioactive.
   C. Keep a shielded container in the room in case a radioactive source is dislodged from the client.
   D. All materials leaving the client's room are surveyed by the radiation safety officer or designee.

ANSWERS

1. *Answer:* A

   Rationale: Radiobiology is the study of events that occur after ionizing radiation is absorbed by living cells. The critical target is believed to be DNA. Repair can occur in both normal and malignant cells. DNA damage may result in cell death, somatic changes, or hereditary changes. A cell injured by ionizing radiation may not demonstrate injury until cell division, which may occur long after the ionizing radiation is absorbed by the cell.

2. *Answer:* B

   Rationale: Cancer cells as well as normal cells vary in their sensitivity to ionizing radiation. Ionizing radiations of comparable types and energies have the same effect on tissue regardless of whether they originate from external beam machines or sealed or unsealed radioactive sources. Hypoxic tissues require higher doses to eradicate cancer cells than do tissues that are well oxygenated. Late responding tissues demonstrate injury as late effects months to years after radiation therapy.

3. *Answer:* D

   Rationale: Fatigue is reported frequently in clients receiving radiation therapy. Treatment of the pelvis may inflame the bladder lining, leading to symptoms of cystitis. When the ovaries are in the radiation field, as in this client, premature menopause is possible. Nausea and vomiting are not likely to be associated with pelvic radiation but are common in abdominal irradiation.

4. *Answer:* C

   Rationale: Strontium 89 is an unsealed radioactive source that cannot be dislodged from the client. It is administered intravenously, thus making all body fluids potentially radioactive. Flushing the toilet three times when urine is disposed of dilutes the radioactivity. Everything that leaves the room is potentially contaminated with radioactivity and must be surveyed before removal.

BIBLIOGRAPHY

Dow, K.H., Bucholtz, J.D., Iwamoto, R., Fieler, V., & Hilderley, L. (eds.). (1997). *Nursing Care in Radiation Oncology* (2nd ed.). Philadelphia: WB Saunders.

Hilderley, L.J., & Dow, K.H. (1996). Radiation oncology. In R. McCorkle, M. Grant, M. Frank-Stromborg, & S. Baird (eds.). *Cancer nursing: A comprehensive textbook* (2nd ed.). Philadelphia: WB Saunders, pp. 331–358.

Hilderley, L.J. (1997). Radiotherapy. In S.L. Groenwald, M.H. Frogge, M. Goodman, & C.H. Yarbro (eds.). *Cancer Nursing: Principles and Practice* (4th ed.). Boston: Jones & Bartlett, pp. 247–282.

Lindsey, A.M., Larson, P.J., Dodd, M.J., Brecht, M., & Packer, A. (1994). Comorbidity nutritional intake, social support, weight and functional status over time in older patients receiving radiotherapy. *Cancer Nurs 17*, 113–124.

Sitton, E. (1997). Nursing implications of radiation therapy. In J.K. Itano & K.N. Taoka (eds.). *ONS Core Curriculum for Oncology Nursing* (3rd ed.). Philadelphia: WB Saunders, pp. 616–629.

Sitton, E.T. (1992). Early and late radiation induced skin alterations: Mechanisms of skin changes (part 1). *Oncol Nurs Forum 19*, 801–808.

Sitton, E.T. (1992). Early and late radiation induced skin alterations: Nursing care of irradiated skin (part 2). *Oncol Nurs Forum 19*, 801–808.

36

Nursing Implications of Biotherapy

Paula Trahan Rieger

Select the best answer for each of the following questions:

1. In the oncology setting, which of the following have not received regulatory approval for the treatment of cancer?
   A. Interferon-alpha.
   B. Monoclonal antibodies.
   C. Effector cells.
   D. Retinoids (tretinoin).

2. Side effects commonly seen with biologic agents such as interferons and interleukins include
   A. thrombocytopenia, neutropenia, and anemia.
   B. flulike symptoms, weight loss, and mucositis.
   C. alterations in mental status, alopecia, and thrombocytopenia.
   D. flulike symptoms, fatigue, and weight loss.

3. Premedications frequently used in the administration of biologic agents include
   A. antiemetics for the control of nausea and vomiting.
   B. steroids to control inflammatory reactions.
   C. acetominophen to control constitutional symptoms.
   D. antidepressants to control mental status changes.

4. Capillary leak syndrome—the movement of fluid from the vascular bed into the tissues—is a frequent side effect seen with the administration of interleukin-2. All of the following are therapeutic interventions to manage this side effect *except*
   A. vasopressors to enhance blood flow to the kidneys and maintain urinary output.
   B. aggressive use of diuretics to promote the elimination of excess fluid.
   C. strict daily weights to monitor accumulation of fluid.
   D. instructing clients to change positions slowly to avoid dizziness.

ANSWERS

1. *Answer:* C

Rationale: Although effector cells are commonly administered in conjunction with interleukin-2 therapy, they remain in investigational status. Interferon-alpha has received regulatory approval for the treatment of hairy cell leukemia, Kaposi's sarcoma, chronic myelogenous leukemia, non-Hodgkin's lymphoma, and as adjuvant therapy for melanoma. Monoclonal antibodies are approved as treatment for lymphoma (rituximab) and breast cancer (trastuzumab). Tretinoin received regulatory approval for the treatment of acute promyelocytic leukemia in 1995.

2. *Answer:* D

Rationale: Side effects commonly seen with the administration of interferons and interleukins include flulike symptoms, fatigue, weight loss related to anorexia, and mental status changes. Thinning of hair versus alopecia is more commonly seen with biologic agents. Although thrombocytopenia, neutropenia, and anemia are seen with the administration of biologic agents, they are not the most commonly experienced side effects and are not experienced to the same degree as in clients receiving chemotherapy and radiotherapy.

3. *Answer:* C

Rationale: Acetominophen should be used as a premedication to control constitutional symptoms, especially in clients receiving interferons and interleukin-2. It may also be used to control bone pain in clients receiving hematopoietic growth factors. Although antiemetics may be used for the administration of interleukin-2, it is not a common intervention for most biologic agents. Steroids are contraindicated with many biologic agents as they may negate the therapeutic effects. Antidepressants are not used as a premedication for mental status changes, which are generally chronic versus acute side effects.

4. *Answer:* B

Rationale: Although diuretics may be used to manage fluid status in clients receiving interleukin-2, they should be used judiciously, not aggressively. The use of vasopressors to maintain urinary output, daily weights, and client education are all appropriate interventions.

BIBLIOGRAPHY

Conrad, K.J., & Horrell, C.J. (eds.). (1995). *Biotherapy: Recommendations for Nursing Course Content and Clinical Practicum.* Pittsburgh: Oncology Nursing Press.

Engelking, C., & Wujcik, D. (1994). Biologic response modifiers (BRMs). In L. Tenenbaum (ed.). *Cancer Chemotherapy and Biotherapy: A Reference Guide* (2nd ed.). Philadelphia: WB Saunders.

Jassak, P.F. (1993). Biotherapy. In S.L. Groenwald, M.H. Frogge, M. Goodman, & C.H. Yarbro (eds.). *Cancer Nursing: Principles and Practice* (3rd ed.). Boston: Jones & Bartlett.

Rieger, P.T. (1998). Nursing implications of biotherapy. In J.K. Itano & K.N. Taoka (eds.). *ONS Core Curriculum for Oncology Nursing* (3rd ed.). Philadelphia: WB Saunders, pp. 630–640.

Rieger, P.T. (ed.). (1996). Biotherapy: Present accomplishments and future projections. *Semin Oncol Nurs* 12(2), 81–171.

Rieger, P.T. (ed.). (1995). *Biotherapy: A Comprehensive Overview.* Boston: Jones & Bartlett.

37

Nursing Implications of Antineoplastic Therapy

Catherine M. Bender

Select the best answer for each of the following questions:

1. Cancer chemotherapy is a systemic form of cancer treatment that is based on concepts of cellular kinetics including the cell life cycle, cell cycle time, growth fraction, and tumor burden. The cell life cycle is
   - A. the length of time required for a cell to move from one mitosis to another.
   - B. the number of cells that are actively dividing in a tumor.
   - C. the process of reproduction that occurs in normal as well as malignant cells.
   - D. the number of cells present in a tumor.

2. Prevention and early detection of extravasation of vesicants or irritants is critical to the safe administration of chemotherapeutic agents. Which of the following is *not* an appropriate intervention for safe administration of chemotherapeutic agents?
   - A. Instruct the client to report any pain or burning experienced during the chemotherapy infusion.
   - B. Administer vesicants in larger veins of the arm, midway between the wrist and elbow.
   - C. Assess for blood return after each l to 2 ml of the chemotherapeutic agent infused.
   - D. Assess for blood return after each 5 to 10 ml of the chemotherapeutic agent infused.

3. Cardiac toxicity is most strongly associated with which of the following chemotherapeutic agents?
   - A. Vincristine.
   - B. Doxorubicin (Adriamycin).
   - C. Nitrogen mustard.
   - D. Cisplatinum.

4. The aim of adjuvant chemotherapy is to
   - A. offset the existence of resistant cells.
   - B. facilitate ease of chemotherapy administration.
   - C. eradicate remaining micrometastases after primary treatment.
   - D. palliate symptoms of clients in whom cure is not possible.

ANSWERS

1. *Answer:* C
   Rationale: The cell life cycle is the process of reproduction that occurs in normal and malignant cells.

2. *Answer:* D
   Rationale: Extravasation can occur with infusion of only 1 to 2 ml of the chemotherapeutic agent.

3. *Answer:* B
   Rationale: Cardiac toxicity is the dose-limiting toxicity of doxorubicin.

4. *Answer:* C
   Rationale: The theoretical goal of adjuvant chemotherapy is to eradicate remaining micrometastases after primary treatment.

BIBLIOGRAPHY

Bender, C.M. (1998). Nursing implications of antineoplastic therapy. In J.K. Itano & K.N. Taoka (eds.). *ONS Core Curriculum for Oncology Nursing* (3rd ed.). Philadelphia: WB Saunders, pp. 641–656.

Bender, C.M., Yasko, J.M., & Strohl, R.A. (1996). Nursing role in management: Cancer. In S.M. Lewis, I.C. Collier, & M.M. Heitkemper (eds.). *Medical-Surgical Nursing: Assessment and Management of Clinical Problems.* St. Louis: Mosby–Year Book, pp. 261–315.

Guy, J.L., & Ingram, B.A. (1996). Medical oncology—the agents. In R. McCorkle, M. Grant, M. Frank-Stromborg, & S.B. Baird (eds.). *Cancer Nursing: A Comprehensive Textbook* (2nd ed.). Philadelphia: WB Saunders, pp. 359–394.

Knobf, M.T., & Durivage, H.J. (1993). Chemotherapy: Principles of therapy. In S.L. Groenwald, M. Goodman, M.H. Frogge, & C.H. Yarbro (eds.). *Cancer Nursing: Principles and Practice* (3rd ed.). Boston: Jones & Bartlett, pp. 270–292.

Krakoff, I.H. (1996). Systemic treatment of cancer. *CA Cancer J Clin 46*(3), 134–141.

Powel, L.L. (ed.). (1996). *Cancer Chemotherapy Guidelines and Recommendations for Practice.* Pittsburgh: Oncology Nursing Press.

Quint-Kasner, S., Chisolm, L., de Carvalho, M., & Piemme, J. (1993). Programmed instruction: Cancer chemotherapy. *Cancer Nurs 16*(1), 63–78.

Wheelock, L.D., & Summers, B.L.Y. (1996). New chemotherapy agents in cancer care. *Oncol Nurs Updates 3*(4), 1–12.

NOTES

38

Principles of Preparation, Administration, and Disposal of Antineoplastic Agents

Jan Hawthorne Maxson and Jean Ellsworth-Wolk

Select the best answer for each of the following questions:

1. ONS Outcome Standards for Chemotherapy Administration were prepared to provide for
   A. safety to personnel, clients, and the environment.
   B. specific procedures for diluting and administering vesicant chemotherapeutic agents.
   C. steps to be followed when administering investigational chemotherapeutic agents.
   D. a mode of evaluating effectiveness of chemotherapeutic agents.

2. The nurse may be exposed to cytotoxic agents by all of the following routes *except*
   A. absorption through skin.
   B. inhalation of aerosols.
   C. direct eye contact.
   D. extravasation of drugs.

3. The appropriate apparel to be worn during administration of chemotherapy according to OSHA guidelines is
   A. disposable gown, goggles, latex gloves, and shoe covers.
   B. disposable gown and latex gloves.
   C. latex gloves and goggles.
   D. disposable gown, shoe covers, and latex gloves.

4. The steps taken following an accidental spill of chemotherapy include all of the following *except*
   A. obtain a spill kit and contain the contaminated area.
   B. wear protective clothing: gloves, gown, shoe covers, and goggles.
   C. wash the contaminated area with diluted bleach solution.
   D. dispose of all contaminated materials in a sealed, thick plastic bag labeled with chemotherapy warning label.

ANSWERS

1. *Answer:* A
   Rationale: Stated in ONS Outcome Standards.

2. *Answer:* D
   Rationale: Extravasation is client exposure. Other responses are all modes of exposure of the nurse.

3. *Answer:* B
   Rationale: OSHA guidelines recommend wearing a disposable, long-sleeved gown made of lint-free fabric with knitted cuffs and a closed front and disposable surgical nonpowdered latex gloves (0.007–0.009 inches) with cuffs long enough to tuck over knit cuffs of gown.

4. *Answer:* C
   Rationale: According to the 1995 OSHA guidelines, the contaminated area is to be washed three times with detergent and rinsed with water.

BIBLIOGRAPHY

American Society of Hospital Pharmacists. (1990). ASHP technical assistance bulletin on handling cytotoxic and hazardous drugs. *Am J Hosp Pharm 47*(15), 1033–1049.

Maxson, J.H., Wolk, J.E. (1998). Principles of preparation, administration, and disposal of antineoplastic agents. In J.K. Itano & K.N. Taoka (eds.). *Core Curriculum for Oncology Nursing* (3rd ed.). Philadelphia: WB Saunders, pp. 657–661.

Oncology Nursing Society. (1996). *Cancer Chemotherapy Guidelines.* Pittsburgh: Oncology Nursing Society.

Occupational Safety and Health Administration. (1995). *OSHA Work Practice Guidelines for Personnel Dealing with Cytotoxic (Antineoplastic) Drugs.* Washington, D.C.: Author.

Tenenbaum, L. (1994). *Cancer Chemotherapy and Biotherapy: A Reference Guide.* Philadelphia: WB Saunders.

NOTES

39

Nursing Implications of Bone Marrow and Stem Cell Transplantation

Robi Thomas

Select the best answer for each of the following questions:

1. Which of the following is *not* a reason for GM-CSF or G-CSF to be used for clients undergoing marrow transplantation?
    - A. Clients may be at decreased risk for veno-occlusive disease.
    - B. Clients may be at decreased risk of infections.
    - C. Graft failure may be reversed.
    - D. Hospital stays may be shortened.

2. Which drug is not used to prevent graft-versus-host disease?
    - A. Cyclosporine A.
    - B. Decadron or prednisone.
    - C. Cytarabine.
    - D. FK-506 (tacrolimus).

3. Which of the following would *not* be an appropriate recipient for an umbilical cord blood transplant?

    - A. A client who is believed to match a family member's cord blood.
    - B. A client who has a match found in the Cord Blood Registry and weighs 50 kg.
    - C. A client who weighs 22 kg who is believed to match a family member's cord blood.
    - D. A client who weighs 90 kg and needs an allogeneic transplant.

4. Which of the following is *not* a sign of acute graft-versus-host disease?
    - A. A macular-papular rash that began on the palms of the hand and soles of the feet.
    - B. Sclerodermic skin changes that began on day 125.
    - C. Increased amounts of diarrhea—up to 3 L/24 h.
    - D. Encephalopathy and increased serum bilirubin levels.

ANSWERS

1. *Answer:* A.
   Rationale: VOD (veno-occlusive disease) is not prevented by the use of growth factors.

2. *Answer:* C.
   Rationale: Cytarabine is a cytotoxic agent. The other three choices are all agents used to prevent graft-versus-host disease.

3. *Answer:* D.
   Rationale: Umbilical cord blood transplants are usually used for clients who weigh less than 60 kg.

4. *Answer:* B.
   Rationale: Sclerodermic skin changes are often a sign of chronic graft-versus-host disease. Acute graft-versus-host disease typically occurs within the first 90 days of transplantation.

BIBLIOGRAPHY

Buchsel, P.C. (1997). Allogeneic bone marrow transplantation. In S. Groenwald, M.H. Frogge, M. Goodman, & C.H. Yarbro (eds.). *Cancer Nursing: Principles and Practice* (4th ed.). Boston: Jones & Bartlett, pp. 459–506.

Smith, B.R. (1997). Stem cell transplantation. In V.T. DeVita, S. Hellman, & S.A. Rosenberg (eds.). *Cancer Principles and Practice of Oncology* (5th ed.). Philadelphia: Lippincott-Raven, pp. 2621–2638.

Wikle-Shapiro, T. (1998). Nursing implications of bone marrow and stem cell transplantation. In J.K. Itano & K.N. Taoka (eds.). *ONS Core Curriculum for Oncology Nursing* (3rd ed.). Philadelphia: WB Saunders, pp. 662–677.

Wujcik, D. (1997). Autologous bone marrow and blood cell transplantation. In S. Groenwald, M.H. Frogge, M. Goodman, & C.H. Yarbro (eds.). *Cancer Nursing: Principles and Practice* (4th ed.). Boston: Jones & Bartlett, pp. 507–526.

NOTES

PART VII

Health Promotion

40

Prevention of Cancer

Sharon J. Olsen

Select the best answer for each of the following questions:

1. Excessive alcohol consumption has been associated with all types of cancer *except*
   A. buccal cavity.
   B. large bowel.
   C. breast.
   D. gallbladder.

2. The *Year 2000 Dietary Objectives* of the National Cancer Institute (NCI) include all the following *except*
   A. decreasing daily consumption of fat from 40% to 25% of total calories.
   B. minimizing consumption of foods preserved by salt-curing.
   C. increasing daily consumption of vitamins A, C, and E.
   D. increasing consumption of fiber from grains, fruits, and vegetables to 20 to 30 g/d.

3. Colon cancer prevention strategy includes which one of the following?
   A. Reduction of red meat in the diet.
   B. Modification of dietary fat intake.
   C. Pursuit of a diet rich in vegetables.
   D. Pursuit of a diet rich in fiber and vegetables.

4. Of all the risk factors that have been associated with the development of cancer, which one of the following is currently believed to be responsible for the greatest number of cancers?

   A. Occupational exposures.
   B. Personal habits or lifestyles.
   C. Environmental exposures.
   D. Congenital and genetic disorders.

5. Obesity has been named as a risk factor for which of the following cancers?
   A. Stomach cancer.
   B. Lung cancer.
   C. Prostate cancer.
   D. Corpus uteri cancer.

6. From a client's history, the nurse discerns the following: the client does not practice breast self-examination regularly, is a heavy coffee drinker, is infected with condyloma acuminatum (HPV), and follows a diet that is high in fat and low in fiber, fruits, and vegetables. Of these risk factors, which one has been clinically linked with a type of cancer?
   A. A diet high in fat and low in fiber and fruits and vegetables.
   B. Physical manipulation of the breast.
   C Caffeine consumption.
   D. Infection with HPV.

7. A triad of risk factors for endometrial cancer is
   A. nulliparity, radiation to pelvic area, and Plummer-Vinson syndrome.
   B. obesity, hypertension, and diabetes mellitus.
   C. Bowen's disease, nulliparity, and long-term use of conjugated estrogens.
   D. higher socioeconomic class, cancer of the breast, and history of menstrual irregularities.

8. Cryptorchidism puts a child at risk for which one of the following cancers?
   A. Leukemia.
   B. Testicular cancer.
   C. Sarcoma.
   D. Wilms' tumor.

9. Cancer risk may be defined as the likelihood that exposure to a certain factor will influence the chance of developing a particular cancer. Three types of risks are commonly used to explain cancer occurrence. Select the incorrect definition:
   A. Absolute risk measures cancer incidence and mortality.
   B. Relative risk measures the excess chance of developing cancer imposed by exposure to a risk factor relative to the risk that may exist without the exposure.
   C. Predictive risk measures the percentage of cancer that can be predicted to occur given a specific exposure to a risk factor.
   D. Attributable risk measures the amount of cancer prevented by eliminating exposure to a risk factor.

10. A comprehensive clinical approach for promoting primary prevention includes
    A. risk assessment.
    B. assessing client's perception of risk.
    C. mutual agreement on intervention.
    D. facilitating and promoting client action.

11. Mechanisms of carcinogenesis predict that cancer may directly result from all of the following *except*
    A. hormonal factors.
    B. poverty.
    C. inherited or acquired alterations in proto-oncogenes or tumor suppressor genes.
    D. occupational and environmental exposures.

12. Tobacco use has been associated with all of the following tumor groups *except*
    A. nasopharynx, oral cavity, throat.
    B. lung, bladder, pancreas.
    C. breast, brain, melanoma.
    D. stomach, cervix, esophagus.

13. The genetic predisposition for cancer is often characterized by a series of cardinal features. Which of the following is *not associated* with familial cancer risk?
    A. Early age of cancer onset.
    B. Tumor unilaterality.
    C. Multiple primary cancers.
    D. Multiple family members with cancer.

14. A 38-year-old woman has a 54-year-old brother in whom hereditary nonpolyposis colorectal cancer (HNPCC) was diagnosed 4 years ago. After 25 years as an inner-city bus driver during which the client smoked at least a pack of cigarettes a day, she has developed bladder cancer. This client could attribute her bladder cancer to all of the following *except*
    A. genetics.
    B. age.
    C. cigarette smoking.
    D. occupational exposure.

15. Which of the following is *not* considered a premalignant condition?
    A. Leukoplakia of the mouth.
    B. Dysplasia of the cervix.
    C. Erythroplakia of the mouth.
    D. Crohn's disease.

16. Individuals who have had an organ transplant are at increased risk for cancer. Which cancer occurs most commonly in transplant clients?
    A. Leukemia.
    B. Hodgkin's disease.
    C. Multiple myeloma.
    D. Non-Hodgkin's lymphoma.

17. Of all the classes of chemotherapy, which class has the strongest potential for carcinogenic activity?
    A. Alkylating agents.
    B. Antimetabolites.
    C. Plant alkaloids.
    D. Antibiotics.

18. Which of the following clinical scenarios illustrates primary prevention for cancer?
    A. A school nurse designs a creative program to encourage teenagers to delay sexual activity as well as practice "safe sex."
    B. A public health nurse receives a grant to purchase a mobile van that will serve low-income housing areas and offer free Papanicolaou smears.

C. An occupational nurse sets up a breast self-examination training program for women in a dress-making factory.

D. A geriatric nurse practitioner receives funding from the Association of Retired Persons to distribute Hemoccult slides to residents of a retirement community.

19. Which of the following triad of risk factors is not associated with colorectal cancer?
   A. High-fat diet, reduced intake of calcium, a low-fiber diet.
   B. A personal history of colorectal adenomas, breast cancer, or ovarian cancer.
   C. High-carbohydrate intake, *Helicobacter pylori* infection, intake of nitrates and smoked foods.
   D. A family history of familial adenomatous polyposis, a personal history of juvenile polyposis, a personal history of chronic ulcerative colitis.

20. Viruses have been implicated in carcinogenesis. Which of the following combinations are likely to be virally initiated?
   A. Non-Hodgkin's lymphoma, pancreatic cancer, and bladder cancer.
   B. Non-Hodgkin's lymphoma, T-cell leukemia, and cervical cancer.
   C. Cervical cancer, T-cell leukemia, and pancreatic cancer.
   D. Hepatocellular cancer of the liver, cervical cancer, and bladder cancer.

21. Lifestyle risk factors include all of the following *except*
   A. tobacco use and diet.
   B. side stream smoke exposure and occupational exposures.
   C. environmental exposures and alcohol intake.
   D. viral exposures and familial/genetic contributions.

22. The director of your state's environmental health program has asked you to consult on the development of a new public health services grant proposal. The purpose of this grant is to significantly reduce the number of cancer deaths related to a select environmental cause. A focus on which of the following could be expected to produce the largest public health impact?
   A. Electromagnetic field (EMF) exposure and childhood cancer.
   B. Cancers of the brain and nervous system and cellular telephone use.
   C. Ultraviolet exposure and skin cancers.
   D. Hazardous waste dump exposure and leukemia.

23. Environmental tobacco smoke (side stream smoke) has been associated with all of the following childhood illnesses *except*
   A. bronchitis and pneumonia.
   B. fluid in the middle ear and reduced lung function.
   C. asthma attacks and respiratory tract irritation.
   D. sore throat and tonsilitis.

24. A nurse has designed an intervention strategy for the primary prevention of colorectal cancer. Appropriate clinical outcomes for this primary prevention intervention would include the client's doing all of the following *except*
   A. identifying colorectal cancer risk factors associated with lifestyle and genetics.
   B. describing the Hemoccult collection procedure and recommendations.
   C. identifying barriers and facilitators to adopting colorectal cancer prevention strategies.
   D. developing a plan for behavior change.

25. Health risk appraisals generate a self-reported, computerized client health profile. They assume that information regarding personal risk factor levels and the benefits of reducing these risk factors will motivate clients to adopt lifestyle changes. The use of health risk appraisals is recommended for mass screening programs, public marketing campaigns, and health fairs. Weaknesses of such surveys include all of the following *except*
   A. they often are based on outdated statistics.
   B. they generally provide no opportunity to assess adherence to recommendations.
   C. reliability and validity are seldom assessed.
   D. they provide no opportunity to clarify myths or misconceptions.

26. The Agency for Health Care Policy and Research (AHCPR) has developed a plan for every health care provider to follow to assist their clients to stop smoking. This plan includes all of the following *except*
    A. ask about and record the tobacco use status of every client.
    B. advise every smoker to quit smoking.
    C. assist the client with a quit plan.
    D. distribute smoking cessation literature at health fairs.

27. All of the following USDA/USDHHS recommendations for daily food group consumption are true *except*
    A. eat 2 to 4 servings of fruit per day.
    B. eat 3 to 5 servings per day of vegetables.
    C. consume 6 to 11 servings of bread, cereal, rice, or pasta each day.
    D. consume one serving of lean meat, skinless poultry, or fish per day.

28. Low serum levels of selenium have been associated with a risk for which of the following cancers?
    A. Breast cancer.
    B. Bladder cancer.
    C. Lung cancer.
    D. Osteosarcoma.

29. Chemoprevention trials with calcium supplements have been associated with a reduction in risk for which of the following cancers?
    A. Colon cancer.
    B. Breast cancer.
    C. Osteosarcoma.
    D. Melanoma.

NOTES

ANSWERS

1. *Answer:* D
   Rationale: Alcohol is a lifestyle risk factor. Many cancer sites can be affected by excessive alcohol intake.

2. *Answer:* C
   Rationale: The *Year 2000 Goals* for the nation include decreasing cancer mortality by 50%. This goal requires health care providers to participate in educating the public. Increasing vitamins is not one of these recommendations. Rather, vitamins can be increased by eating more fruits and vegetables. Diet is a lifestyle risk factor for cancer.

3. *Answer:* D
   Rationale: A diet high in fiber and vegetables promotes regular excretion of stool.

4. *Answer:* B
   Rationale: Lifestyle factors are responsible for the greatest number of cancers and are the most amenable, though difficult, to change.

5. *Answer:* D
   Rationale: Obesity is a lifestyle risk factor that is significant in corpus uteri cancer.

6. *Answer:* D
   Rationale: HPV is a virus that has been directly linked with, but not proven as a single cause of, carcinoma of the cervix. Sexual activity is a lifestyle risk factor.

7. *Answer:* B
   Rationale: Endometrial cancer is one of the leading cancers in older women. There is a definite triad of risk factors associated with this cancer. These are personal risk factors.

8. *Answer:* B
   Rationale: Cryptorchidism is a personal risk factor that places the child at increased risk for testicular cancer.

9. *Answer:* C
   Rationale: Epidemiologic research has enabled health care providers to identify individuals and populations that may be at increased risk of developing cancer. Attention to these risks facilitates the targeting of appropriate cancer control interventions to individuals at increased risk for developing cancer. There is no such thing as predictive risk.

10. *Answer:* B
    Rationale: A, C, and D are process variables associated with promoting behavioral change. B is a psychosocial variable associated with the internal motivation for changing behavior.

11. *Answer:* B
    Rationale: At this time, there is no evidence that poverty directly contributes to carcinogenesis.

12. *Answer:* C
    Rationale: Tobacco use accounts for about 30% of all cancer deaths. This lifestyle risk factor is a known contributor to cancers of the lung, bladder, pancreas, cervix, esophagus, oral cavity, stomach, nasopharynx, and throat.

13. *Answer:* B
    Rationale: Inherited genetic mutations account for 5% to 10% of all cancer cases. Bilaterality, the presence of cancer in twin organs such as the eyes (retinoblastoma) or the breasts (breast cancer), for example, is an important characteristic of familial cancer.

14. *Answer:* B
    Rationale: Risk factors associated with bladder cancer include occupational exposure to exhaust fumes, a family history of HNPCC, and a history of cigarette smoking. Most cancers occur after the age of 50 years; age is not a significant contributor in this particular case.

15. *Answer:* D
    Rationale: Premalignant conditions predispose the individual to cancer. All choices except D are classified as premalignant conditions and as lifestyle risk factors are amenable to prevention.

16. *Answer:* D
    Rationale: This is an example of an iatrogenic risk factor. Clients are at increased risk of cancer because of medical treatments.

17. *Answer:* A
    Rationale: Alkylating agents, known chemical carcinogens, have the greatest potential for producing a second malignancy. Recognition of this iatrogenic risk factor has nursing implications for long-term follow-up and regular screening.

18. *Answer:* A
    Rationale: The question requires that the nurse differentiate between primary and secondary prevention of cancer. Responses B, C, and D are examples of screening or detection programs.

19. *Answer:* C
    Rationale: The risk factors listed under C are associated with a risk for gastric cancer not colorectal cancer.

20. *Answer:* B
    Rationale: Viral exposures may account for up to 15% of cancers. Viral exposures have been linked to hepatocellular carcinoma of the liver, Kaposi's sarcoma (HIV), non-Hodgkin's lymphoma (EBV), cervical cancer (HPV), and T-cell leukemia (HTLV-1)

21. *Answer:* D
    Rationale: All factors listed in A, B, and C are considered lifestyle related. Viral exposures and familial/genetic contributions are considered to be biologic risk factors.

22. *Answer:* C
    Rationale: Environmental risk factors contribute to only about 2% of all cancer deaths. However, sunlight exposure, in particular ultraviolet (UV) B exposure, contributes to about 90% of skin cancers including melanoma. A statewide campaign to reduce sun exposure could significantly affect the number of skin cancer deaths.

23. *Answer:* D
    Rationale: As much as 30% of all lung cancers not associated with tobacco smoking may be attributed to environmental tobacco smoke exposure. Children living in homes with one or more smoking adults have been found to have increased rates of bronchitis, pneumonia, middle ear infections, respiratory tract infections, and asthma.

24. *Answer:* B
    Rationale: Outcomes A, C, and D are all appropriate for primary prevention. Outcome B concerns secondary prevention (screening).

25. *Answer:* C
    Rationale: The usefulness of health risk appraisals has been criticized broadly in the literature. These population-based surveys provide aggregate data with little opportunity to connect interventions with clinical outcomes. Such appraisals are, however, frequently assessed for reliability and validity.

26. *Answer:* D
    Rationale: The AHCPR's recommendations include points A, B, and C. Also, the nurse should act as a role model by not smoking and follow-up client to counsel for relapse or reinforce abstinence.

27. *Answer:* D
    Rationale: 2 to 3 servings of meat and meat alternatives are recommended. Also recommended are 2 to 3 servings of milk, yogurt, or cheese per day; 3 to 6 servings of fats; avoidance of sweets and moderate alcohol intake; limited consumption of salt-cured, smoked, and nitrite-preserved foods.

28. *Answer:* C
    Rationale: Clinical trials of selenium supplements have found protective effects for cancers of the lung, colon, rectum, and prostate.

29. *Answer:* A
    Rationale: Calcium supplements have been found to reduce hyperproliferation of the colonic mucosa cells, thereby providing a protective effect against colon cancer.

BIBLIOGRAPHY

Greenwald, P., Kramer, B.S., & Weed, D.L. (1995). *Cancer Prevention and Control.* New York: Marcel Dekker.

Olsen, S.J., & Frank-Stromborg, M. (1996). Cancer screening and early detection. In R. McCorkle, M. Grant, M. Frank-Stromborg, & S.B. Baird (eds.). *Cancer Nursing: A Comprehensive Textbook.* Philadelphia: WB Saunders, pp. 265–297.

Olsen, S.J., Morrison, C.H., & Ashley, B.W. (1998). Prevention of cancer. In J.K. Itano & K.N. Taoka (eds.). *ONS Core Curriculum for Oncology Nursing* (3rd ed.). Philadelphia: WB Saunders, pp. 681–694.

41

Screening and Early Detection of Cancer

Candis H. Morrison

Select the best answer for each of the following questions:

1. Cancer screening tests are used to
   A. titrate chemotherapy dosage in clients with a known cancer diagnosis.
   B. follow progression of disease through subsequent examinations.
   C. diagnose symptomatic individuals.
   D. identify asymptomatic persons with risk factors for cancer.

2. The prevalence of any disease is defined as
   A. the number of cases, both old and new, present at a point in time in a defined population.
   B. the number of new cases during a specified period in a defined population.
   C. the number of deaths attributed to the disease during a specified period in a defined population.
   D. the number of persons among all those who have a form of the disease and die of it during a specified period.

3. When consideration is being given to whether a screening program is warranted based on characteristics of the population to be screened, all of the following require consideration *except* whether
   A. the prevalence of the disease in the population is sufficiently high.
   B. the population is accessible to the screening program.
   C. the population is likely to comply with the recommended diagnostic tests and treatment.
   D. there is no effective treatment available for the disease.

4. Which statement is *true* regarding the selection bias of a screening test? It
   A. can occur if clients undergoing screening have better health habits than the general population.
   B. reflects the fact that at any point in time the population will include persons with aggressive disease.
   C. occurs when disease is detected earlier but the detection does not affect mortality.
   D. gives the appearance of improved survival in screen-detected cases because the diagnosis is moved forward by screening; however, it merely lengthens the interval from diagnosis to death, rather than lengthening life.

5. Client assessment always requires a thorough history. Which of the following statements is true of the history of present illness (HPI)?
   A. It is a concise statement regarding the client's reason for the visit.
   B. A complete symptom analysis is mandatory.
   C. It uses the occupational risk assessment tool.
   D. It reviews *all* body systems for potential complaints that could possibly be related to cancer.

6. Socioeconomic status (SES) is a demographic variable that requires consideration when a risk profile ratio is being developed for a client. All the following are reasons to include this data *except*
   A. There is greater tobacco use among poorer populations.
   B. Low SES groups avail themselves of screening services less often.
   C. Urbanization and pollution are associated with decreased incidences of disease.
   D. Rural and lower SES groups present with more advanced disease.

7. A finding of concern when examining the female breast is
   A. bilateral inverted nipples.
   B. a unilateral inverted nipple.
   C. bilateral ptosis.
   D. unilateral accessory nipple.

8. The triad of currently recommended breast cancer screening modalities is best reflected in which of the following sets?
   A. Mammography, ultrasonography, surgical consultation.
   B. Ultrasonography, magnetic resonance imaging, computed tomography.
   C. Ultrasonography, fine-needle aspiration (FNA), and cytopathology.
   D. Mammography, clinical breast examination, and breast self-examination.

9. Rectal examinations in asymptomatic clients over 40 include all of the following *except*
   A. inspection for external lesions, masses.
   B. palpation for masses.
   C. color of rectal mucosa.
   D. stool for occult blood.

10. The most significant information one can obtain from a digital prostate examination is the assessment of
   A. rectal sphincter tone.
   B. consistency and size of prostate gland.
   C. mucosal composition of prostate tissue.
   D. prostatic atrophy.

11. Pap smear screening has life-saving potential because
   A. cervical carcinoma progresses rapidly in most women.
   B. carcinoma in situ (CIS) persists in the detectable state for an extended time before becoming invasive.
   C. CIS is readily detectable by a serum marker.
   D. Pap smears remove layers of carcinoma-involved tissue and thus lessen the chance of disease progression.

12. Which of the following is *not* a rationale for performing fecal occult blood tests in eligible or symptomatic individuals?
   A. Serum tests are superior to stool blood markers, as they have no dietary prohibitions.
   B. Many colon cancers lie beyond the reach of standard sigmoidoscopies.
   C. Many more colon cancers are being detected in the right colon these days.
   D. Stool blood testing can help detect cancer or polyps in asymptomatic individuals.

13. When providing dietary instruction for individuals undergoing fecal occult blood testing (FOBT), it is important to stress that
   A. intake of foods high in peroxidase activity (turnips and broccoli) should be increased.
   B. multivitamins with iron are permitted.
   C. acetaminophen is a pain reliever that will not interfere with testing.
   D. vitamin C is permitted.

14. As a serum marker, prostate specific antigen (PSA)
   A. is specific for prostate cancer.
   B assists in diagnosis of rectal carcinoma as well as prostate.
   C. is a glycoprotein produced by most prostate carcinomas.
   D. is recommended for all males over 30 years of age.

15. Breast self-examination (BSE) should be performed
   A. every year in women over age 20.
   B. every month, one week after the onset of menses in women over 20.
   C. by all women starting at age 40.
   D. after any breast symptom becomes problematic.

16. In asymptomatic individuals age 40 or above, with what frequency do the American Cancer Society Guidelines recommend that health counseling and cancer check-ups be performed?
    A. Every year.
    B. Every three years.
    C. Every five years.
    D. At the onset of a sign or symptom of cancer.

17. Secondary prevention emphasizes
    A. the use of various diagnostic tests to rule out or confirm the presence of disease in asymptomatic persons.
    B. the regular, ongoing monitoring of persons who have already been identified as high risk.
    C. the clinical problem-solving process applied to clients with abnormal screening tests.
    D. early diagnosis and prompt treatment to halt the pathologic process.

18. Endometrial biopsy is recommended in
    A. every woman who is sexually active.
    B. postmenopausal women who complain of vaginal bleeding.
    C. women in whom human papilloma virus is suspected.
    D. women with a history of herpes simplex virus.

19. The *best* current use of the PSA test is to provide data for
    A. screening asymptomatic individuals.
    B. evaluation of normal prostatic tissue growth.
    C. disease recurrence.
    D. diagnosis of prostatic cancer.

20. Screening recommendations for cervical cancer include
    A. baseline and annual human choriogonadotropin (hCG) levels.
    B. annual clinical examination beginning at the onset of menarche.
    C. Papanicolaou (Pap) smear every 1 to 3 years in women over the age of 20 or with the onset of sexual activity.
    D. Pap smear at the time of any evidence of sexually transmitted disease.

21. Which of the following statements is *true* regarding pelvic examinations in women after menopause?
    A. If there have been three consecutively negative Pap smears, pelvic examination is not necessary on a yearly basis.
    B. Pelvic examinations are required every year even if Pap smears are not.
    C. Negative Pap smears effectively rule out ovarian carcinoma.
    D. Positive Pap smears raise suspicion of ovarian carcinoma.

22. The American Cancer Society does *not* recommend screening for which one of the following cancers?
    A. Lung cancer.
    B. Cervical cancer.
    C. Oral cancer.
    D. Colorectal cancer.

23. Which one of the following screening practices has been demonstrated to be the *most* effective in reducing cancer mortality?
    A. Yearly chest x-ray examinations and sputum cytology for lung cancer.
    B. Monthly skin self-examination.
    C. Pap smears at least once every 3 years for women between 20 and 70.
    D. Monthly testicular examination.

24. A screening test with high sensitivity yields
    A. few false negatives.
    B. many false negatives.
    C. few false positives.
    D. many false positives.

25. Colorectal screening recommendations do *not* include
    A. fecal occult blood testing in persons over the age of 50.
    B. sigmoidoscopy in persons over the age of 50.
    C. fecal occult blood testing for fiber intolerance.
    D. periodic colonoscopy for familial polyposis syndrome history.

26. In the TNM staging system the T portion reflects which of the following?
    A. Time of onset of the tumor.
    B. Time tumor is biopsied in relation to its onset.
    C. The extent of the primary tumor.
    D. The presence of metastatic dissemination.

27. All of the following are useful techniques to lower barriers to early cancer detection *except*
   A. teach and monitor self-examination procedures.
   B. personalize recommendations based on individual history and risk profiles.
   C. target high-risk groups.
   D. use only highly sensitive tests.

28. The rationale for the development of risk profiles and screening guidelines is to
   A. enhance screening efficacy and decrease costs.
   B. promote uniform staging.
   C. provide an estimate of the burden of the disease in a defined population.
   D. improve the sensitivity and specificity of screening tests.

NOTES

ANSWERS

1. *Answer:* D

   Rationale: There are three categories of laboratory tests: screening tests, diagnostic tests, and tests used in the management of clients. Screening tests are used to identify asymptomatic persons with risk factors for disease, detect occult disease and permit early treatment, reassure clients found free of disease with or without risk factors, and provide genetic counseling in familial conditions. A and B are descriptions of tests used in the management of clients, and C is used for diagnosis, not screening.

2. *Answer:* A

   Rationale: These epidemiologic principles assist in the study of the distribution and determinants of disease in population groups and assist in the development of population-based risk profiles. The B response is actually a definition of incidence; C defines mortality; and D defines case fatality.

3. *Answer:* D

   Rationale: A, B, and C are characteristics of the population that can be used to determine if a screening program is warranted. D is incorrect because screening will not be of benefit if there is no effective treatment.

4. *Answer:* A

   Rationale: If the clients screened have healthier behaviors than the general population, they will have a lower incidence of all diseases in which lifestyle is a contributing factor, e.g., smoking and lung cancer, sun exposure and skin cancer. The remainder of the selections do not describe selection bias.

5. *Answer:* B

   Rationale: Any symptom requires a detailed comprehensive analysis based on onset, location, duration, characteristics, aggravating and relieving factors, and timing. The A response is a definition of the chief complaint. The C response belongs under the occupational history section. The D response is true of the review of systems section of the comprehensive health history.

6. *Answer:* C

   Rationale: Urbanization and pollution are associated with *increased* incidences of disease, not decreased. Tobacco use is higher, use of screening services is lower, and disease at presentation is more advanced in lower SES populations.

7. *Answer:* B

   Rationale: This is particularly true if this is a new finding. Bilateral inverted nipples are a normal variant if not a recent change. Bilateral ptosis is a normal effect of aging. Unilateral accessory nipples, also called supernumerary nipples are a common finding, especially in African Americans.

8. *Answer:* D

   Rationale: Ultrasonography is used to differentiate solid from cystic masses. Magnetic resonance imaging, FNA, and cytopathology are reserved for diagnostic, not screening purposes.

9. *Answer:* C

   Rationale: A, B, and D are components of a rectal examination. Color of rectal mucosa cannot be determined without additional equipment such as an anoscope, which is not part of the examination in asymptomatic clients.

10. *Answer:* B

    Rationale: Although determining rectal sphincter tone is important in a rectal examination, the main purpose of performing a prostate examination is to check for size, nodularity, and firmness or hardness of the gland. Prostatic atrophy is not a disease entity, and mucosal composition can only be determined microscopically.

11. *Answer:* B

    Rationale: Because CIS persists in a detectable state for a long time, the Pap smear is an appropriate and effective screening tool. A is incorrect because cervical carcinoma is *not* a rapidly progressing disease in most women. C is incorrect because there is currently no serum marker for CIS. D is incorrect, as removal of superficial cervical and endocervical cells does not affect disease progression.

12. *Answer:* A

    Rationale: There are no serum markers to

measure fecal blood loss. Hematocrit or hemoglobin level may drop late in disease, so they are not adequate early detection tests. B, C, and D *are* rationales for performing fecal occult blood tests as part of a screening evaluation.

13. *Answer:* C
Rationale: Pain relievers such as aspirin and other NSAIDs may cause occult gastrointestinal bleeding and thus a positive test. Iron, vitamin C, and certain vegetables (particularly turnip family) cause false positive FOBT results.

14. *Answer:* C
Rationale: A is incorrect because PSA is also elevated in other more common conditions such as benign prostatic hypertrophy. B is not true, as rectal carcinoma is diagnosed through digital rectal examination, FOBT, and sigmoidoscopy. D is inaccurate as PSA is not used in men between 30 and 40 years of age.

15. *Answer:* B
Rationale: BSE should be performed monthly, 1 week after the onset of menses in all women over age 20. A and C are therefore incorrect responses. D is incorrect because BSE is proposed to detect breast symptoms before they become problematic.

16. *Answer:* A
Rationale: Cancer checkups are recommended annually in asymptomatic persons over 40. In persons under 40 they are recommended every 3 years. D is incorrect, as the evaluation is diagnostic after the onset of a sign or symptom of cancer.

17. *Answer:* D
Rationale: Response A is a component of early primary detection, not secondary prevention. Response B defines surveillance. Response C defines diagnosis. D is the only choice that is encompassed by the term "secondary prevention."

18. *Answer:* B
Rationale: Women with unexpected (non-hormone-replacement-related) postmenopausal bleeding should be evaluated for endometrial hyperplasia, which is a precursor to endometrial cancer. Every woman who is sexually active needs Pap smear screening. Human papilloma and herpes virus may cause cervical dysplasia and are therefore rationales for frequent Pap screening.

19. *Answer:* C
Rationale: PSA is a biochemical marker for prostate cancer. Levels are used to follow disease progression. Levels will rise if there is a recurrence after treatment. Because of its lack of specificity, use of PSA for screening purposes is controversial. Diagnosis requires tissue for cytopathology.

20. *Answer:* C
Rationale: The American Cancer Society (ACS) recommends a Pap smear every 3 years after two negative tests 1 year apart in women over the age of 20 and in women younger than 20 who are sexually active.

21. *Answer:* B
Rationale: Pelvic examinations are required yearly to check ovary size and consistency. A palpable ovary in a postmenopausal woman raises suspicion of ovarian carcinoma and requires further evaluation. Pap smears are not used to diagnose or rule-out ovarian carcinoma.

22. *Answer:* A
Rationale: The ACS does not recommend routine screening for lung cancer, as there are no currently recommended screening tests for the early detection of this disease that have been shown to make a difference in mortality. Since lung cancer is the leading cause of death from cancer, nurses need to understand that primary prevention, such as smoking cessation, is crucial to reduce the morbidity and mortality of this disease.

23. *Answer:* C
Rationale: Pap smears have been proven to reduce mortality through early detection of cervical carcinoma. Although logically early detection should decrease mortality for most cancers, definitive evidence is strongest for Pap smears.

24. *Answer:* A
Rationale: Sensitivity is defined as a measure of the probability that a test result will be positive if the disease being investigated is present. The fewer false negatives, the more sensitive the test. A test with 100% sensitivity will always be positive in the presence of the disease it tests for.

25. *Answer:* C

Rationale: Responses A and B correspond with the ACS guidelines for the asymptomatic population. Familial polyposis of the colon is an inherited autosomal dominant trait and is a personal risk factor for colon cancer. People with a family history of this disease require close follow-up. Fiber intolerance does not require testing for fecal occult blood.

26. *Answer:* C

Rationale: Responses A and B are not part of the staging system, and D reflects the M portion.

27. *Answer:* D

Rationale: Highly sensitive tests will not lower barriers to early detection as the other options do. Highly sensitive tests will produce few false negative results but do not actually affect detection barriers.

28. *Answer:* A

Rationale: The other choices are not rationales for risk profiles and screening guidelines. Staging and test sensitivity and specificity are irrelevant, whereas choice C describes an aspect of prevalence.

BIBLIOGRAPHY

Davis, M. (1992). Secondary prevention in oncology nursing practice. In J.C. Clark & R.F. McGee (eds.). *ONS Core Curriculum for Oncology Nursing* (2nd ed.). Philadelphia: WB Saunders, pp. 46–61.

Mettlin, C., Jones, G., Averette, H., et al. (1993). Defining and updating the American Cancer Society guidelines for the cancer-related checkup: Prostate and endometrial cancers. *CA Cancer J Clin 43*(1), 42–46.

Reintgen, D.S., & Clark, R.A. (eds.). (1996). *Cancer Screening.* St. Louis: Mosby–Year Book.

Tilkian, S.M., Conover, M., & Tilkian, A.G. (eds.). (1995). *Clinical and Nursing Implications of Laboratory Tests.* St. Louis: Mosby–Year Book.

NOTES

PART VIII

Professional Performance

42

Application of the Standards of Practice and Education

Deborah Lowe Volker

Select the best answer for each of the following questions:

1. The American Nurses Association (ANA)/ Oncology Nursing Society (ONS) *Standards of Oncology Nursing Practice* can be used to do all of the following *except*
   A. develop a conceptual framework for cancer nursing education programs.
   B. assist in the development of performance evaluation tools.
   C. develop institution-specific client care standards.
   D. meet Joint Commission on the Accreditation of Healthcare Organizations (JCAHO) standards.

2. The 11 high-incidence problem areas in oncology nursing cited in the ANA/ONS *Standards of Oncology Nursing Practice* are
   A. key areas in which oncology nurses assess, plan, and intervene.
   B. problems that most often affect the client in the acute care setting.
   C. clinical indicators that are measurable dimensions of the quality of client care.
   D. the problems with the highest incidence rates.

3. The oncology nurse evaluates his or her own nursing practice in relation to professional practice standards and relevant statutes and regulations. Which of the following statements reflects

a *measurement criterion* that indicates this standard was met? The oncology nurse
   A. shares knowledge and skills with colleagues and others during practice.
   B. seeks regular, constructive feedback regarding own practice and role performance from peers, professional colleagues, clients, and others.
   C. collaborates with other health care providers in educational programs and consultation, management, and research endeavors as opportunities arise.
   D. evaluates factors related to safety, effectiveness, and cost when two or more practice options would result in the same expected client outcome.

4. The oncology nurse identifies expected outcomes individualized to the client. Which of the following measurement criteria supports this standard? The oncology nurse
   A. incorporates preventive, therapeutic, rehabilitative, palliative, and comforting nursing actions into the plan of care.
   B. reviews and revises the nursing diagnoses, expected outcomes, and plan of care based on the findings of the evaluation process.
   C. communicates the client's responses with the health care team.
   D. ensures that expected outcomes provide direction for continuity of care.

5. An intended outcome of the ONS *Standards of Oncology Education: Patient/Family and Public* is to
   A. delineate strategies for teaching tool development.
   B. improve consistency and accuracy of information included in patient teaching.
   C. improve health promotion and care for the public.
   D. provide guidelines for content.

6. Personal behaviors and public policy related to cancer prevention, detection, control, rehabilitation, and supportive care are influenced by formal and informal cancer public education. Which of the following indicates achievement of this standard?
   A. Public education programs include signs and symptoms of common cancers.
   B. An environment conducive to learning is maintained.
   C. The oncology nurse provides leadership in the development of public education materials.

D. The public reached by cancer education participates in cancer-screening activities.

7. Before teaching a patient about prevention and early detection of colorectal cancer, the nurse should
   A. help the client identify personal risk factors for colorectal cancer.
   B. discuss the need to comply with screening activities.
   C. evaluate the client's readiness to learn.
   D. assess the client's normal bowel patterns.

8. To validate education materials for use in culturally diverse populations, the oncology nurse should
   A. submit materials to a group of hospital volunteers for review.
   B. seek input from representative members of the populations.
   C. ask community leaders to review the materials.
   D. conduct a survey using a random sample of clients.

NOTES

ANSWERS

1. *Answer:* D
   Rationale: The *Standards* define the scope of cancer nursing practice and, as such, should form the basis for oncology nursing programs, including clinical practice, education, administration, and research. They do not specify how to meet JCAHO standards.

2. *Answer:* A
   Rationale: The 11 high-incidence areas refer to clinical problems that oncology clients most often experience, regardless of the care setting.

3. *Answer:* B
   Rationale: Although all four options are measurement criteria for the *Standards of Professional Performance,* choice B is the only one that pertains to performance appraisal.

4. *Answer:* D
   Rationale: According to the ANA/ONS *Standards,* D supports the outcome standard. A supports planning; B supports evaluation; and C supports implementation.

5. *Answer:* C
   Rationale: The *Standards* provide guidelines for the development, implementation, and evaluation of client-teaching and public education programs.

6. *Answer:* D
   Rationale: According to the ONS *Standards*

the public reached by cancer education will participate in screening activities.

7. *Answer:* C
   Rationale: Teaching-learning theories dictate that effective teaching is based on an assessment of the client's readiness to learn, learning needs, and situational and psychosocial factors influencing learning.

8. *Answer:* B
   Rationale: Only answer B specifically includes representatives from the groups in question. The other methods do not ensure representatives from all cultural subgroups in a population.

BIBLIOGRAPHY

Dorsett, D.S. (1993). Quality of care. In S.L. Groenwald, M.H. Frogge, M. Goodman, & C.H. Yarbro (eds.). *Cancer Nursing: Principles and Practice* (3rd ed.). Boston: Jones & Bartlett, pp. 1453–1484.

Iwamoto, R., Rumsey, K., & Summers, B. (1996). *Statement on the Scope and Standards of Oncology Nursing Practice.* Washington, DC: American Nurses Publishing.

Miaskowski, C., & Rostad, M. (1990). Implementing the ANA/ONS Standards of Oncology Nursing Practice. *J Nurs Qual Assur* 4(3), 15–23.

Oncology Nursing Society. (1995). *Standards of Oncology Education: Patient/Family and Public.* Pittsburgh: Author.

Volker, D.L. (1998). Application of the standards of practice and education. In J.K. Itano & K.N. Taoka (eds.). *Core Curriculum for Oncology Nursing* (3rd ed.). Philadelphia: WB Saunders, pp. 713–726.

43

The Education Process

Mary B. Johnson

Select the best answer for each of the following questions:

1. A 48-year-old woman is discharged following a lumpectomy for a newly diagnosed malignant breast tumor. She is to have radiation therapy following incision healing. Which of the following depicts the most appropriate nursing diagnosis category and etiology for this woman?
   A. Active role in health maintenance related to surgery (lumpectomy).
   B. Knowledge deficit related to mastectomy.
   C. Risk for anxiety related to knowledge deficit of breast cancer treatment.
   D. Pain related to breast cancer and mastectomy.

2. The overall purpose of the educational component of nursing practice is to help people acquire the knowledge they need to
   A. comply with the physicians' orders.
   B. learn what health professionals believe they need to know.
   C. understand their particular diagnosis.
   D. participate in their own decisions and self-care.

3. The nurse prepares an educational plan for a client who is about to receive chemotherapy for colon cancer. The client is a professor of political science at a large university and is eager to carry on with his work. Which of the following statements represents a learning principle that would be especially important for this client?
   A. Learning should be subject centered not client centered.

B. Learner-identified needs should receive priority.
C. Learning is often negated by life experiences.
D. Learning occurs when the teaching plan is completed.

4. The nurse is in charge of developing an education program for clients who are starting their first regimen of chemotherapy. To evaluate the success of the presentation it is necessary to identify expected outcomes. Which of the following statements would represent an appropriate expected outcome for this program? Upon completion of this educational program the client will be able to
   A. describe strategies for managing common side effects of chemotherapy.
   B. understand the role of chemotherapy in cancer treatment.
   C. learn about community resources available for cancer care.
   D. know the names of the chemotherapy drugs he or she is taking.

5. Participation in cancer-related public education is an important nursing activity because
   A. these programs have potential impact on cancer prevention, incidence, morbidity, and mortality.
   B. these programs enhance the professional image of cancer nursing.
   C. the participants' fear of cancer will be modified.
   D. the competence of the nurse as a cancer-client educator will improve.

6. Mr. Anderson had a hemicolectomy with colostomy 2 days ago. In assessing his readiness for attending a 15-minute teaching session on ostomy care, you would be most interested in
    A. his educational level.
    B. his comfort level.
    C. his ability to walk.
    D. his socioeconomic status.

7. Staff education is defined as employer-sponsored activities and experiences aimed at expanding and improving professional performance in order to
    A. improve staff satisfaction.
    B. increase the educational level of the staff.
    C. meet Joint Commission on the Accreditation of Healthcare Organizations (JCAHO) standards.
    D. improve client, family, and community health outcomes.

8. Which of the following emotional states increase a client's receptivity to learning?
    A. Mild anxiety.
    B. Medications that control physical responses.
    C. Fatigue.
    D. Fever.

NOTES

ANSWERS

1. *Answer:* C
   Rationale: Etiologies consist of behaviors of the client, or factors in the environment, or an interaction of both. A medical diagnosis is not considered appropriate because it does not individualize the cause of the problem. Knowledge deficit is most appropriately used as an etiology in this case because it is a risk factor for anxiety.

2. *Answer:* D
   Rationale: The overall purpose of client education is to enable full participation, acceptance of responsibility, and shared decision making. Compliance often implies instructions that the client is expected to obey. Client education focuses on empowering the individual for self-care.

3. *Answer:* B
   Rationale: Learning occurs when a person perceives a need to learn something; therefore learner-identified needs should receive priority. Learning should be problem centered, is influenced by accumulated life experiences, and may not be accomplished even with instruction.

4. *Answer:* A
   Rationale: A well-stated, expected outcome identifies a behavior or an action that the learner will be able to do. Understanding, learning, and knowing are not actions and are difficult to measure.

5. *Answer:* A
   Rationale: Participation in public cancer-related programs is believed to positively affect cancer prevention and detection activities and ultimately cancer morbidity and mortality.

6. *Answer:* B
   Rationale: Physical responses that alter comfort can decrease motivation and receptiveness to learning.

7. *Answer:* D
   Rationale: Although meeting JCAHO standards and improving staff satisfaction may be important, the ultimate focus of staff education is on improving the health outcomes of clients, families, and the community. JCAHO standards address client-focused care.

8. *Answer:* A
   Rationale: Physical responses that alter comfort, such as fatigue and fever, and medications that control physical responses decrease motivation and receptiveness to learning. Research indicates that mild or moderate anxiety may be helpful to learning.

BIBLIOGRAPHY

American Nurses Association/Oncology Nursing Society. (1996). *Standards of Oncology Nursing Practice.* Washington, DC: American Nurses Association.

Carpenito, L.J. (1993). *Handbook of Nursing Diagnosis* (5th ed.). Philadelphia: JB Lippincott, pp. 8–11.

Rankin, S., & Stallings, K. (1996). *Patient Education: Issues, Principles, and Practices* (3rd ed.). Philadelphia: JB Lippincott, pp. 5, 14–15, 21–40, 99–118, 135, 157, 321.

Oncology Nursing Society. (1995). *Standards of Oncology Education: Patient/Family and Public.* Pittsburgh: Author, pp. 4–13.

44

Legal Issues Influencing Cancer Care

Mary Magee Gullatte

Select the best answer for each of the following questions:

1. Which of the following professional sources provides the nurse with a mechanism for due process and penalties?
   A. American Nurses Association Standards of Practice.
   B. Oncology Nursing Society Standards of Practice.
   C. Nurse Practice Act.
   D. American Society of Clinical Oncology Standards.

2. The liability issue in nursing practice concerned with the care relationship between client and provider is referred to as
   A. duty.
   B. negligence.
   C. malpractice.
   D. breach of duty.

3. In deciding which source affects legal decision making as it relates to agency or institutional policies and procedures, the nurse should know that
   A. institutional policies override regulations.
   B. regulations override institutional policies.
   C. standards override regulations.
   D. regulations override statutes.

4. The nurse is monitoring a client on a morphine drip. The nurse enters the pump to clear a kink in the tubing. The clamp is left open and the drug free flows into the client. This would be an example of which of the following liabilities?

   A. Duty.
   B. Negligence.
   C. Malpractice.
   D. Breach of duty.

5. A nurse enters the room of a client who is receiving intravenous chemotherapy. The nurse checks the bag and infusion rate. When reviewing the label she finds that the bag hanging is labeled with another client's name and is not the right drug. Legally the nurse who hung the wrong drug has committed which of the following?
   A. Negligence.
   B. Malpractice.
   C. Duty.
   D. Breach of duty.

6. Which client agreement should be initiated if a client requests a Do Not Resuscitate order?
   A. Durable power of attorney.
   B. Living will.
   C. Patient rights.
   D. Medical ethics.

7. Which of the following patient rights organizations actively protects the constitutional rights of citizens?
   A. People's Medical Society.
   B. American Society of Law and Medicine.
   C. American Civil Liberties Union.
   D. National Health Law Program.

8. You are planning a discharge for a client with terminal cancer. The client tells you that she is tired of fighting and "just wants it to end."

She asks you to refer her to an organization that can offer her support. You would most appropriately recommend which one of the following organizations?

A. Hemlock Society.
B. National Hospice Society.
C. People's Medical Society.
D. American Civil Liberties Union.

NOTES

ANSWERS

1. *Answer:* C

Rationale: The Nurse Practice Act provides definition and role of nursing by state. It regulates the practice of professional nursing and provides a mechanism for due process and penalties.

2. *Answer:* A

Rationale: Duty addresses the care relationships between the client and provider.

3. *Answer:* B

Rationale: Regulations are rules of conduct set by local, state, or federal government and override institutional policies.

4. *Answer:* B

Rationale: In this scenario the nurse was negligent in not following the acceptable standard of care in managing intravenous therapy, care that a reasonable person would give in a specific situation.

5. *Answer:* D

Rationale: In this case the nurse failed to meet the acceptable standard of care, which would have been to follow the "5 Rs" of medication administration, which was the wrong client.

6. *Answer:* B

Rationale: This written agreement is initiated by the client prior to or while accessing the health care environment to document his or her wishes in the event of cardiac or respiratory arrest.

7. *Answer:* C

Rationale: The ACLU actively protects the rights of citizens conferred by the Constitution.

8. *Answer:* B

Rationale: Information center about hospices, which would be the most appropriate support for this terminal cancer client.

BIBLIOGRAPHY

Annas, G.J. (1992). *The Rights of Patients: The Basic ACLU Guide to Patient Rights* (rev. ed.). Carbondale, IL: Southern Illinois University Press.

Barhamand, B.A. (1996). Documentation issues in cancer nursing. In R. McCorkle, M. Grant, M. Frank-Stromborg, & S. Baird (eds.). *Cancer Nursing: A Comprehensive Textbook.* Philadelphia: WB Saunders, pp. 1356–1365.

Hall, J.K. (1996). *Nursing Ethics and Law.* Philadelphia: WB Saunders.

Hoefler, J.M. (1994). *Deathright: Culture, Medicine, Politics, and the Right To Die.* Boulder, CO: Westview Press.

McCabe, M.S., & Piemme, J.A. (1996). Cancer legislation. In R. McCorkle, M. Grant, M. Frank-Stromborg, & S. Baird (eds.). *Cancer Nursing: A Comprehensive Textbook.* Philadelphia: WB Saunders, pp. 1356–1365.

Scanlon, C., & Fibison, W. (1995). *Managing Genetic Information: Implications for Nursing Practice.* Washington, DC: American Nurses Publishing.

Stromborg, M.F., & Chamorro, T. (1996). Legal responsibilities of the nurse. In R. McCorkle, M. Grant, M. Frank-Stromborg, & S. Baird (eds.). *Cancer Nursing: A Comprehensive Textbook.* Philadelphia: WB Saunders, pp. 1356–1365.

45

Selected Ethical Issues in Cancer Care

Rose Mary Padberg

Select the best answer for each of the following questions:

1. The main purpose of informed consent in clinical trials is to
   A. enable autonomous choice.
   B. protect the client against harm.
   C. ensure responsible medical and nursing actions.
   D. increase accrual in clinical trials.

2. Mrs. B. is not sure about signing the informed consent for her therapy. The nurse is eager to enroll Mrs. B. in the study. In her zeal to recruit for this study, the nurse must be especially careful to maintain the ethical principle of
   A. veracity.
   B. autonomy.
   C. beneficence.
   D. justice.

3. Traditionally children, prisoners, the mentally impaired, and the elderly have been considered "vulnerable populations." This is because they often
   A. lack control of their life situation.
   B. may be susceptible to coercion by those in authority over them.
   C. may not have the cognitive ability to make an autonomous choice.
   D. all of the above.

4. Medical paternalism is viewed as a violation of the ethical principle of
   A. justice.
   B. autonomy.

C. veracity.
D. beneficence.

5. Mrs. M. has told you that she does not intend to read the informed consent document before her chemotherapy. She said it was too upsetting. What is your best response?
   A. You need to read the document before we can start the treatments.
   B. Let's go over it together. We can discuss the parts that may be upsetting you.
   C. Let me get the doctor and we can decide what to do.
   D. Chemotherapy is risky, but you need to sign the document before we can proceed.

6. Mr. H. has lung cancer and has been given several options for treatment. He is unsure of what to do and asks you, "What would you do?" Your best answer would be
   A. I would choose the treatment with the best response rate.
   B. I have seen many clients do well on the cisplat regimen.
   C. The decision is up to you.
   D. I can see how making a decision about which treatment to choose can be difficult. Let's talk about the options.

7. The role of the nurse regarding a durable power of attorney for health care is to
   A. educate the client regarding the opportunity to establish durable power of attorney for health care.
   B. refer the client to appropriate resources for information.

C. promote communication between the health care team and the person holding the durable power of attorney for health care.

D. all of the above.

8. The specialty of oncology nursing presents many ethical dilemmas regarding life-sustaining treatment efforts. When questions arise involving the use or the removal of extraordinary means of life support, it may be helpful to consult which one of the following groups for guidance?

    A. Institutional Review Board (IRB).

    B. Hospital ethic's committee.

    C. Hospital lawyer.

    D. All of the above.

NOTES

ANSWERS

1. *Answer:* A
   Rationale: The purpose of informed consent is to assist the client in making an informed choice regarding the upcoming therapy. Increasing accrual to a clinical trial is not the purpose of the consent form.

2. *Answer:* B
   Rationale: Clients must make treatment decisions based on information that is factual, unbiased, and noncoercive.

3. *Answer:* D
   Rationale: These populations are vulnerable to exploitation and coercion because of their lack of autonomy. Great care must be taken to protect their rights and safety.

4. *Answer:* B
   Rationale: Paternalism assumes the decision-making function for another person; thus autonomous choice is not possible.

5. *Answer:* B
   Rationale: Clients need to be aware of what to expect regarding the risks, benefits, and alternatives of the chemotherapy treatments. When the risks have been discussed, the client can make an informed choice about whether to have the treatments. Having an informed client is also having a client who will be aware of what to expect and how to manage it.

6. *Answer:* D
   Rationale: Encourage questions and provide nondirective counseling to assist the client in making a decision. Assume the role of client advocate and assist the client to come to his or her best choice.

7. *Answer:* D
   Rationale: A durable power of attorney in health care legally designates an individual who is responsible for making health care decisions on behalf of a person who is no longer competent or able to do so.

8. *Answer:* B
   Rationale: An objective third party often can be of great assistance in helping the family and the health care professionals weigh the moral issues and arguments of the proposed intervention and come to a thoughtful resolution.

BIBLIOGRAPHY

Faden, R.R., & Beauchamp, T.L. (1986). *A History and Theory of Informed Consent.* New York: Oxford University Press.

Vanderpool, H.Y. (1996). *The Ethics of Research Involving Human Subjects: Facing the 21st Century.* Frederick, MD: University Publishing Group.

Veatch, R.M. (1997). *Medical Ethics.* Boston: Jones & Bartlett.

46

Cancer Economics and Health Care Reform

Mary Ann Crouch

Select the best answer for each of the following questions:

1. Managed care promotes the following concepts
   A. Linkage of provider systems, cost containment and utilization, maintaining quality and access.
   B. Disassociation of providers, increased use of physician extenders, increased access to health.
   C. Fixed reimbursement, control of costs, maintaining quality.
   D. Linkage of provider systems, control of costs, maintaining quality.

2. The focus of health care delivery in a managed care plan is
   A. continuity of care.
   B. episodic treatment.
   C. liberal provider autonomy.
   D. strict control over the use of specialists.

3. A DRG is
   A. a mechanism to decide admission to a hospital.

   B. a standard used to determine the expected length of hospitalization for a particular diagnosis.
   C. a system developed to determine reimbursement for inpatient hospitalization specific to diagnosis.
   D. a system to evaluate utilization of hospital services.

4. Examples of legislative interventions developed to contain health care costs include
   A. DRGs, Medicaid expansion, supply cost-control.
   B. clinical pathways, treatment guidelines.
   C. financial information systems.
   D. universal access to health care.

5. Evidence that suggests the cost of cancer care will continue to escalate includes
   A. expensive new cancer drug developments.
   B. expanding aged population.
   C. increased reimbursement for clinical research.
   D. increased Medicaid expenses.

ANSWERS

1. *Answer:* A
   Rationale: Managed care is defined as the linkage of payers, providers, and purchasers in systems and activities that control costs and utilization of care while maintaining high quality and access.

2. *Answer:* A
   Rationale: Managed care promotes continuity of care rather than episodic treatment.

3. *Answer:* C
   Rationale: DRG (diagnosis related group) is a system of Medicare classification for inpatient hospital services based on primary and secondary diagnoses, procedures, age, sex, and complications. DRGs are used as a financing mechanism to reimburse hospitals and providers for services rendered.

4. *Answer:* A
   Rationale: DRGs, Medicaid expansion, and supply cost-control are strategies developed to manage health care costs at the state and national level. Clinical pathways and treatment guidelines remain focused at the practitioner or organizational level, as do financial systems.

5. *Answer:* B
   Rationale: Age continues to be the greatest risk for developing cancer, and the percentage of elderly adults continues to increase as we approach the year 2000. Elderly clients with cancer demonstrate special needs related to treatment and management of complications and side effects.

BIBLIOGRAPHY

Antman, K. (1993). Reimbursement issues facing patients, providers, and payers. *Cancer 72*(suppl), 2842–2845.

Antman, K., Berkman, B.J., Huber, S.L., et al. (1993). The economic impact of therapy on cancer patients. *Cancer 72*(suppl), 2862–2849.

Brown, M.L., & Fireman, B. (1995). Evaluation of direct medical costs related to cancer. *J Natl Cancer Inst 87,* 399–400.

Coile, R.C. (1992). Health care outlook 1995: Strategic directions for oncology. *J Oncol Manage 1*(15), 31–33.

Goldsmith, J.C., Goran, M.J., & Nackel, J.G. (1995). Managed care comes of age. *Health Care Forum J 38*(5), 14–24.

Jenks, S. (1995). Some HMO's embrace clinical trials. *J Natl Cancer Inst 87,* 1104.

Kennedy, B.J. (1994). Oncology issues in health care reform. *Cancer Invest 12,* 249–256.

Leake, A.R. (1995). The economic impact of cancer. *Nurse Pract Forum 6,* 207–214.

Smith, T.J., Hilner, B.E., & Desch, C.E. (1993). Efficacy and cost-effectiveness of cancer treatment: Rational allocation of resources based on decision analysis. *J Natl Cancer Inst 85,* 1460–1474.

47

Changes in Oncology Health Care Settings

Ellen Carr

Select the best answer for each of the following questions:

1. The client's health care coverage has become the dominant influencing factor in
   A. first line chemotherapy protocols.
   B. access to health care.
   C. the client's selection of power of attorney.
   D. the decision to participate in support groups.

2. Successful ambulatory care for oncology clients requires all of the following *except*
   A. a collaborative approach to client management.
   B. client and family participation in care.
   C. general symptom management.
   D. appropriate age-related education materials.

3. Issues in oncology rehabilitation are a primary focus of the following programs *except*

A. Look Good, Feel Good.
B. The International Association of Laryngectomies.
C. American Association of Retired Persons—AARP.
D. I Can Cope.

4. The primary responsibility of the home care nurse is to
   A. provide 24-hour on-call support.
   B. collaborate with the primary care physician.
   C. teach the proper use of medications.
   D. support the primary caregiver.

5. The hospice care setting that relies on the home as the place of care is a
   A. community-based program.
   B. hospital-based program.
   C. associated oncology practice.
   D. free-standing hospice.

ANSWERS

1. *Answer:* B
Rationale: Access to health care is dictated by the measurable outcome of cost-effective quality care and is determined by the client's health care coverage.

2. *Answer:* C
Rationale: Symptom management needs to be customized to the client's individual needs.

3. *Answer:* C
Rationale: The AARP is an advocacy group addressing issues affecting seniors and the elderly. Cancer rehabilitation is not the primary focus of the organization.

4. *Answer:* D
Rationale: The home care nurse guides and augments care provided by the primary caregiver(s).

5. *Answer:* A
Rationale: Community-based hospices rely on the client's family, friends, and community volunteers to support care.

BIBLIOGRAPHY

Beddar, S.M., & Aiken, J.L. (1994). Continuity of care: A challenge for ambulatory oncology nursing. *Semin Oncol Nurs 10*(4), 254–263.

Berry, D.E., Boughton, L., & McNamee, F. (1994). Patient and physician characteristics affecting the choice of home based hospice, acute care inpatient hospice facility, or hospitals as last site of care for patients with cancer of the lung. *Hosp J 9*(4), 21–38.

Boyle, D.M. (1994). New identities: The changing profile of patients with cancer, their families and their professional caregivers. *Oncol Nurs Forum 21*(1), 55.

Cooley, M.E., Lin, E.M., & Hunter, S.W. (1994). The ambulatory oncology nurse's role. *Semin Oncol Nurs 10*(4), 245–253.

Dudgeon, D.J., Raubertas, R.F., Doerner, K., et al. (1995). When does palliative care begin? A needs assessment of cancer patients with recurrent disease. *J Palliat Care 11*(1), 5–9.

Ferrell, B., & O'Neil-Page, E. (1993). Continuity of care. In S.L. Groenwald, M.H. Frogge, M. Goodman, & C. Yarbro (eds.). *Cancer Nursing: Principles and Practice* (3rd ed.). Boston: Jones & Bartlett, p. 1346.

Frymark, S., & Mayer, D. (1993). Rehabilitation of the person with cancer. In S.L. Groenwald, M.H. Frogge, M. Goodman, & C. Yarbro (eds.). *Cancer Nursing: Principles and Practice* (3rd ed.). Boston: Jones & Bartlett, p. 1360.

Harvey, C. (1994). New systems: The restructuring of cancer care delivery and economics. *Oncol Nurs Forum 21*(1), 72–77.

Varricchio, C. (1994). Human and indirect costs of home care . . . for cancer patients. *Nurs Outlook 42*(4), 151–157.

Walter, J. (1994). Nursing care delivery models in ambulatory oncology. *Semin Oncol Nurs 10*(4), 237–244.

48

Professional Issues in Cancer Care

Coni Ellis

Select the best answer for each of the following questions:

1. Continued professional competency can be achieved through all of the following methods *except*
   A. continuing education.
   B. client reviews.
   C. annual performance appraisals.
   D. periodic refresher courses.

2. Groups that collaborate successfully share the following characteristic:
   A. a common, articulated sense of purpose.
   B. open communication, including expression of opposing views.
   C. a flexible decision-making process.
   D. all of the above.

3. Collaboration between industry and clinical sites fosters research and improves client care. The key to successful collaboration is that
   A. all products are provided free to the clinical site.
   B. negotiated agreements spell out responsibilities.
   C. industry provides the specific protocol to be followed.
   D. clinical sites complete all data collection and analysis.

4. Characteristics within the workplace that contribute to stress or burnout include all of the following *except*
   A. decreased use of nurse registries and unlicensed personnel.
   B. limited opportunity to participate in decision making.
   C. inappropriate discharges.
   D. overcrowded units, noise, malfunctioning equipment.

5. Concrete strategies for coping with stress include
   A. establishing a sense of control over one's practice.
   B. compartmentalizing life and work.
   C. acknowledging vulnerabilities.
   D. all of the above.

6. Organizational support for oncology nursing is promoted by which of the following activities?
   A. Sexual harassment policies and procedures.
   B. Stop the violence programs.
   C. Recognition and financial incentives.
   D. All of the above.

7. Peer review is a process in which professional nurses appraise the quality of care provided by professional nurse(s) in accordance with established standards. These standards may be found in all of the following *except*
   A. Joint Commission on Accreditation of Health Care Organizations (JCAHO).
   B. Occupational Safety and Health Agency (OSHA).
   C. state nurse practice acts.
   D. professional literature.

8. A nurse who conveys a client's needs and concerns to the client's physician is practicing which type of advocacy?

A. Consumer advocacy.
B. Paternalistic advocacy.
C. Simplistic advocacy.
D. Consumer-centric advocacy.

9. After a nurse clarifies a procedure for a client, the client decides he does not want to have it. The nurse supports the client by informing the physician of the client's decision. Indicate the type of advocacy.

A. Simplistic advocacy.
B. Consumer-centric advocacy.
C. Paternalistic advocacy.
D. Consumer advocacy.

NOTES

ANSWERS

1. *Answer:* C
   Rationale: Annual performance appraisals may be biased by the evaluator, and criteria used may not address clinical competencies. They are often completed by persons who do not actually observe the actual performance of the person.

2. *Answer:* D
   Rationale: All these criteria are identified by Steel as necessary for successful collaboration.

3. *Answer:* B
   Rationale: For collaboration to be successful, all parties involved need to be included in the negotiations, and each party's responsibilities need to be specified in the agreement.

4. *Answer:* A
   Rationale: In an effort to achieve more cost-effective staffing practices, institutions have increased use of temporary-help agencies and unlicensed personnel, which often has led to more stress for the regular staff because the temporary personnel are not familiar with the institution's procedures and delegating tasks once done by RNs to unlicensed personnel creates dilemmas.

5. *Answer:* D
   Rationale: All these actions lead to setting boundaries that would enable one to cope with stress.

6. *Answer:* D
   Rationale: In today's workplace federal law mandates that employers provide protection for all employees with regard to sexual harassment and violence. Changes in economic forces are now affecting job satisfaction, and therefore stress can be reduced through planned monetary and recognition incentives.

7. *Answer:* B
   Rationale: The Occupational Safety and Health Agency (OSHA) is responsible for developing regulations that promote the safety and health of workers. It does not address standards of client care.

8. *Answer:* C
   Rationale: Simplistic advocacy is the act of one pleading for the cause of another.

9. *Answer:* B
   Rationale: Consumer-centric advocacy is the act of a nurse providing a client with information and then supporting the client in his decision.

BIBLIOGRAPHY

Abruzzese, R. (1996). Nursing staff development/strategies for success. In P. Yoder Wise (ed.). *Learning Needs Assessment.* St. Louis: Mosby–Year Book, pp. 188–207.

Abruzzese, R. (1997). Nursing staff development/strategies for success. In J.M. Katz & E. Green (eds.). *Managing Quality: A Guide to System-wide Performance Management in Health Care* (2nd ed.). St. Louis: Mosby–Year Book, pp. 302–324.

Abruzzese, R. (1996). Nursing staff developments/strategies for success. In C.A. Mottola (ed.). *Research in Nursing Staff Development.* St. Louis: Mosby–Year Book, pp. 326–344.

American Nurses Association and Oncology Nursing Society. (1996). *Standards of Oncology Nursing Practice.* Washington, DC: American Nurses Publishing.

American Nurses Association. (1995). *Nursing: A Social Policy Statement.* Washington, DC: American Nurses Publishing.

American Nurses Association. (1989). *Education for Participation in Nursing Research.* Washington, DC: American Nurses Publishing.

Baranoski, B., Reil, L., Vogt, N., McIntosh, A., Rahen, E., Weaver, M.C., & Rosenzweig, M. (1995). Nursing and industry: A time for collaboration. *Adv Wound Care* 8(2), 46–52.

Ellis, C. (1998). Professional issues in cancer care. In J.K. Itano & K.N. Taoka (eds.). *Core Curriculum for Oncology Nursing* (3rd ed.). Philadelphia: WB Saunders, pp. 770–791.

Fitzpatrick, M.J. (1994). Performance improvement through quality improvement teamwork. *J Nurs Admin* 24(12), 20–27.

Gaydon, J.E., West, P., Galloway, S., et al. (1993). Bridging the gap between research and clinical practice: A collaborative approach. *Oncol Nurs Forum* 20(6), 953–957.

Greco, K.E. (1995). Regulation of advanced nursing practice: Part II. Certification. *Oncol Nurs Forum* 22(8), 39–42.

Hogston, R. (1995). Nurses' perceptions of the impact of continuing professional education on the quality of nursing care. *J Adv Nurs* 22(3), 86–93.

Joint Commission on Accreditation of Healthcare Organizations. (1996). *Accreditation Manual for Hospitals.* Chicago: Author.

King, J.M., White, M.A., Buckwalter, K.C., Whall, A., Lederman, R., Speer, J., Lasky, P., & McLane, A. (1985). A group dynamics view. *West J Nurs Res 7*, 7–19.

Kircholl, K.T., & Mateo, M.M. (1996). Roles and responsibilities of clinical nurse researchers. *J Prof Nurs 12*(2), 86–90.

Lazarus, R. (1996). *Psychological Stress and the Coping Process.* New York: McGraw-Hill.

Manion, J. (1995). Understanding the seven stages of change. *Am J Nurs 95*(6), 41–43.

McCaffrey Boyle, D. (1994). New identities: The changing profile of patients with cancer, their families, and their professional caregivers. *Oncol Nurs Forum 21*(1), 55–60.

McCaffrey Boyle, D., Engelking, C., & Harvey, C. (1994). Are oncology nurses ready? *Oncol Nurs Forum 21*(1), 53–55.

McCaffrey Boyle, D., Engelking, C., & Harvey, C. (1994). Taking command of the future: Getting ready now for the 21st century. *Oncol Nurs Forum 21*(1), 77–79.

McGuire, D.F., Walczak, J.P., & Krum, S.C. (1994). Development of a nursing research utilization program in a clinical oncology setting: Organization, implementation, and evaluation. *Oncol Nurs Forum 21*(4), 704–709.

Oncology Nursing Society. (1995). *ONS Standards of Oncology Nursing Education: Generalist and Advanced Practice Levels.* Pittsburgh: Oncology Nursing Press.

Pritchett, P., & Pound, R. (1995). *A Survival Guide to the Stress of Organizational Change.* Dallas: Pritchett and Associates.

Rafael, A. (1995). Advocacy and empowerment: Dichotomous or synchronomous concepts? *Adv Nurs Sci 18*(2), 25–32.

Reiley, P., Seibert, C.P., Miller, N.E., et al. (1994). Implementation of a collaborative quality assessment program. *J Nurs Admin 24*(5), 65–71.

Steel, J. (1986). *Issues in Collaborative Practice.* Orlando, FL: Grune & Stratton.

NOTES

49

Issues and Challenges: Alternative Therapies

Paul J. Ross

Select the best answer for each of the following questions:

1. Persons most likely to embrace alternative therapies include which of the following?
   A. Well-educated cosmopolitan persons.
   B. Immigrants.
   C. Economically disadvantaged persons.
   D. The likelihood for all is the same.

2. Alternative therapies are best understood as
   A. practices that oppose conventional medicine and, consequently, encourage noncompliance.
   B. practices that often are used in conjunction with biomedical interventions and consequently cause minimal health risk.
   C. a broad range of practices outside of conventional medicine that claim physiological benefit often without significant empirical bases.
   D. generally noninvasive practices that offer hope and encouragement to clients and consequently should be respected and supported.

3. Alternative practices are best distinguished from conventional therapies by which of the following? They
   A. use benign "natural" products or less invasive procedures.
   B. are based on a body of knowledge that is often informally shared and that is not part of nursing and medical school curricula.
   C. rely on evidence of efficacy that is more often anecdotal and less frequently subject to scientific scrutiny.

   D. utilize interventions that generally exclude pharmacologic and physiologic treatment.

4. All of the following alternative and complementary therapies are being increasingly incorporated into mainstream cancer programs *except*
   A. healing touch.
   B. immunoaugmentative therapy.
   C. osteopathy.
   D. traditional healing techniques guided by native healers.

5. When discussing alternative therapies with clients, the nurse should remember that the appeal of many therapies includes all of the following *except*
   A. an approach that is often holistic and personal.
   B. an understanding of pathology and physiology that is jargon free and easy to understand.
   C. an explanation that is inherently logical.
   D. a promise of cure that clients seek.

6. The oncology nurse can assist clients interested in alternative therapies by
   A. encouraging open communication about biomedical options and alternative or complementary therapies.
   B. emphasizing the proven value of biomedical options.
   C. reporting evidence of alternative therapy use to attending physicians.
   D. recommending that clients first give biomedicine a chance before exploring alternative strategies.

ANSWERS

1. *Answer:* D

   Rationale: Alternative therapies have a broad-based appeal. Recent investigations identified significant interest in alternative therapies among well-educated, urban, and middle-class clients. These findings have helped to fuel a perspective on alternative therapy that is significantly broader than the one that typically has focused on the isolated practices of a marginal clientele.

2. *Answer:* C

   Rationale: C provides a perspective that is the least value laden and emphasizes the need for more systematic and informed investigations. Option A excludes complementary practices; option B ignores the possible interactions of biomedicines with complementary practices; and option D implies that critical education and appraisal may not be an appropriate intervention.

3. *Answer:* C

   Rationale: Many alternative therapies borrow piecemeal from biomedicine or include controversial (and often expensive) pharmacologic approaches that allegedly target the immune system (e.g., antineoplaston enzyme and amino acid infusions). A serious problem is that many of these practices claim efficacy without proper substantiation. Although efforts have been limited, the National Institutes of Health (NIH) and other research institutions have started to subject these practices to further scientific scrutiny. Likewise, given the popularity of these practices and the potential challenges they present for delivering optimal health care, courses in alternative health are increasingly incorporated into nursing and medical school curricula.

4. *Answer:* B

   Rationale: Immunoaugmentative therapy, designed to target the immune system, is a highly controversial approach of questionable efficacy. The others are increasingly being offered as practices that complement more conventional biomedical approaches.

5. *Answer:* D

   Rationale: Recent evidence suggests that alternative therapies are adopted as much for symptom relief as for cure. There is also ample evidence to indicate that alternative therapies draw adherents because they are effectively communicated. The oncology nurse needs to keep this in mind when trying to meet educational objectives.

6. *Answer:* A

   Rationale: Quick dismissal of alternatives may shut down further communication. Communication necessarily must be nonjudgmental but also informed: nurses must be familiar with the professional and popular literature concerning alternative therapies and be able to discuss alternatives clearly from a biomedical perspective (one that addresses theory and tested outcomes). Option B is likely to shut down further communication. Option C delegates and does not address the question. Option D is based on the assumption that nonconventional practices are secondary interventions to be considered only after biomedicine has failed to meet clients' needs. This either/or approach ignores the often complementary role of alternative therapies or the possibility that clients may have needs that are not completely addressed by biomedicine.

BIBLIOGRAPHY

Burton Goldberg Group. (1994). *Alternative Medicine.* Washington, DC: Future Medicine Publishing.

Cassidy, C. (1996). Cultural context of complementary and alternative medical systems. In M.S. Micozzi (ed.). *Fundamentals of Complementary and Alternative Medicine.* New York: Churchill Livingstone, pp. 9–34.

Cassileth, B.R., & Chapman, C.C. (1996). Alternative and complementary cancer therapies. *Cancer 77*(6), 1026–1034.

Eisenberg, D. (1997). Advising patients who seek alternative medical therapies. *Ann Intern Med 127,* 61–69.

Ernst, E. (1996). The ethics of complementary medicine. *J Med Ethics 22,* 197–198.

Ford, S., Fallowfield, L., & Lewis, S. (1996). Doctor-patient interactions in oncology. *Social Science and Medicine 42*(11), 1511–1519.

Hildenbrand, G., Hildenbrand, L.C., Bradford, K., & Cavin, S.W. (1995). Five-year survival rates of melanoma patients treated by diet therapy after the manner of Gerson: A retrospective review. *Alternative Therapies 1*(4), 29–37.

King, C. (1997). Alternative cancer therapies. In R. Mc-Corkle, M. Grant, M. Frank-Stromborg, & S. Baird (eds.). *Cancer Nursing* (2nd ed.). Philadelphia: WB Saunders, pp. 531–545.

Lane, I.W., & Comac, L. (1996). *Sharks Still Don't Get Cancer.* Garden City Park, NY: Avery Publishing Group.

Lerner, M. (1996). *Choices in Healing. Integrating the Best of Conventional and Complementary Approaches to Cancer.* Cambridge, MA: MIT Press.

Montbriand, M.J. (1995). Decision tree model describing alternative health care choices made by oncology patients. *Cancer Nurs 18*(2), 104–107.

Moss, R.W. (1995). *Cancer Therapy.* New York: Equinox Press.

Nelson, W. (1998). Alternative cancer treatments. *Highlights Oncol Pract 15,* 85–93.

Nwoga, I.A. (1994). Traditional healers and perceptions of the causes and treatment of cancer. *Cancer Nurs 17*(6), 470–478.

Ross, P.J. (1998). Issues and challenges: Alternative therapies. In J.K. Itano & K.N. Taoka (eds.). *Core Curriculum in Oncology Nursing* (3rd ed.). Philadelphia: WB Saunders, pp. 792–795.

Sawyer, M.G., Gannoni, A.F., Toogood, I.R., et al. (1994). The use of alternative therapies by children with cancer. *Med J Australia 160,* 320–322.

Vincent, C., & Furnham, A. (1997). *Complementary Medicine. A Research Perspective.* Chichester, England: John Wiley & Sons.

Youngkin, E., & Israel, D. (1996). A review and critique of common herbal alternative therapies. *Nurse Practitioner 21,* 39–61.

Zaloznik, A.J. (1994). Unproven (unorthodox) cancer treatments. *Cancer Pract 2*(1), 19–24.

ON-LINE REFERENCES

Alternative Medicine Homepage, Falk Library of Health Sciences, University of Pennsylvania. www.pitt.edu/~cbw/alt.html

Office of Alternative Therapy (OAM). www.altmed.od.nih.gov/oam/

Oncolink, University of Pennsylvania Cancer Center. www.oncolink.upenn.edu/specialty/alternative/

Quackwatch. www.quackwatch.com

Richard and Hinda Rosenthal Center of Complementary & Alternative Medicine, Columbia University, College of Physicians & Surgeons. www.cpmcnet.columbia.edu/dept/rosenthal/About_RHRC.html

NOTES